APPLYING QUALITY MANAGEMENT IN HEALTHCARE

APPLYING QUALITY MANAGEMENT IN HEALTHCARE

A Systems Approach

Third Edition

Diane L. Kelly

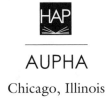

AUPHA

Chicago, Illinois

Your board, staff, or clients may also benefit from this book's insight. For more information on quantity discounts, contact the Health Administration Press Marketing Manager at (312) 424-9470.

This publication is intended to provide accurate and authoritative information in regard to the subject matter covered. It is sold, or otherwise provided, with the understanding that the publisher is not engaged in rendering professional services. If professional advice or other expert assistance is required, the services of a competent professional should be sought.

The statements and opinions contained in this book are strictly those of the author and do not represent the official positions of the American College of Healthcare Executives, the Foundation of the American College of Healthcare Executives, or the Association of University Programs in Health Administration.

Reprinted August 2014

Library of Congress Cataloging-in-Publication Data

Kelly, Diane L.
  Applying quality management in healthcare : a systems approach /
Diane L. Kelly. — 3rd ed.
    p. cm.
  ISBN 978-1-56793-376-5 (alk. paper)
  1. Medical care—Quality control.   2. Health services administration.   3. Total quality management.   I. Title.
  RA399.A1K455   2011
  362.1068—dc22

                                                                    2010054503

The paper used in this publication meets the minimum requirements of American National Standard for Information Sciences—Permanence of Paper for Printed Library Materials, ANSI Z39.48-1984. ∞™

Acquisitions editor: Eileen Lynch; Project manager: Helen-Joy Lynerd; Cover designer: Gloria Chantell; Layout: BookComp

Found an error or a typo? We want to know! Please e-mail it to hap1@ache.org, and put "Book Error" in the subject line.

For photocopying and copyright information, please contact Copyright Clearance Center at www.copyright.com or at (978) 750-8400.

Health Administration Press
A division of the Foundation
  of the American College of
  Healthcare Executives
One North Franklin Street, Suite 1700
Chicago, IL 60606-3529
(312) 424-2800

Association of University Programs
  in Health Administration
2000 North 14th Street
Suite 780
Arlington, VA 22201
(703) 894-0940

To Dan, Anna, and Isabella

BRIEF CONTENTS

DETAILED CONTENTS

FOREWORD

As this book goes to press, the 2010 Patient Protection and Affordable Care Act is the law of the land. Whether the law continues in its present form or is significantly modified in the months and years ahead remains a question. What is not a question is that the issues of quality and the challenges of quality improvement remain a central concern to healthcare providers and those involved with the development of health policy at all levels of our society.

Dr. Diane Kelly in this third edition of *Applying Quality Management in Healthcare* continues to clearly present underlying principles and the fundamentals of quality management and improvement within a systems framework relevant to clinicians and managers in a healthcare setting. The presentation is detailed and focused on the operational realities with specific exercises to develop and fine-tune the skills necessary to meet the challenges of quality management. Some years ago in his role as the president and CEO of the Institute for Healthcare Improvement, Don Berwick described preparing clinicians and managers for the challenges of quality management to be like preparing mountain climbers, and he emphasized the importance of learning the difference between methods and results. In mountain climbing, the focus must be on the basic methods: "how to walk and how to breathe." Healthcare managers and clinicians, like mountain climbers, need to learn the difference between methods and results. This book is about basic methods; it presents real-life quality improvement challenges to provide the reader with the skills necessary to identify goals and vision, define the problem, and apply tools that will influence the results in the same manner as "learning how to walk and breathe" prepares the mountaineer to successfully reach the summit. In quality management as with mountain climbing, the skillful application of the fundamentals is absolutely necessary and needs to be practiced with great discipline. However, if we have learned anything since quality improvement has come of age over the past 40 years, we know that the fundamentals are necessary but not sufficient. While progress is being made, 10 years have passed since the Institute of Medicine published its landmark studies *Crossing the Quality Chasm* (2001) and *To Err is Human* (1999) and at least 30 years since The Joint Commission launched the *Agenda for Change*. Healthcare organizations, clinicians, and those responsible for management and policy decisions are well aware of the underlying concepts of quality management, a great deal of effort and money have been allocated to the cause, and yet, as described by Robert Brook (2010), "there is insufficient evidence about whether or how the quality of care has actually improved." For example, a recent study documented that little change occurred in patient 'harms' during a 6-year review (from 2002 to 2007) of over 2,300 admissions in 10 hospitals in North Carolina, a state and a set of hospitals chosen for study because North Carolina had shown a high level of engagement in patient safety efforts (Landrigan et al. 2010).

Where do we go from here? The systems perspective and fundamentals presented to achieve quality in this third edition need to be internalized by clinicians and managers not as an add-on but as the way we do business, as part of the normal operating procedures of the organization. In addition, their application needs to be viewed within the context of what Don Berwick and colleagues termed "the triple aim" (Berwick, Nolan, and Whittington 2008). That is, "The US will not achieve high value healthcare unless improvement initiatives [interventions] pursue a broader system of linked goals." The triple aim includes

1. to improve the individual experience of care;
2. to improve the health of the population; and
3. to reduce the per capita cost of care for populations.

Clearly the opportunities are at the intersection of these goals. As quality improvement moves forward in an ever-increasingly complex world of cost, expanding technology, and growing expectations, the guidance provided by Dr. Kelly and this third edition proves critical for preparing clinicians and managers to meet the challenges of providing high-value healthcare.

Arnold D. Kaluzny, PhD
Professor Emeritus of Health Policy and Management
UNC Gillings School of Global Public Health
and
Senior Research Fellow
Cecil G. Sheps Center for Health Services Research
University of North Carolina at Chapel Hill

References

Berwick, D. M., T. W. Nolan, and J. Whittington. 2008. "The Triple Aim: Care, Health, and Cost." *Health Affairs* 27 (1): 759–69.

Brook, R. 2010. "The End of the Quality Improvement Movement: Long Live Improving Value." *JAMA* 304 (16): 1831–32.

Landrigan, C. P., G. J. Parry, C. B. Bones, A. D. Hackbarth, D. A. Goldmann, and P. J. Sharek. 2010. "Temporal Trends in Rates of Patient Harm

Resulting from Medical Care." *New England Journal of Medicine* 363 (22) 2124–34.

Institute of Medicine (IOM). 2001. *Crossing the Quality Chasm: A New Health System for the 21st Century.* Washington, DC: National Academies Press.

———. 1999. *To Err Is Human: Building a Safer Health System,* edited by L. T. Kohn, J. M. Corrigan, and M. S. Donaldson. Washington, DC: National Academies Press.

PREFACE

The days when quality was the passion of a select few are gone. The persistence of regulatory, consumer, and clinical leaders has transformed the expectations in all sectors and settings in which health services are offered. The focus has evolved from hospital care to include integration across the continuum of care; from individual patient outcomes to population and community outcomes; from delivering a quality service to ensuring patient safety and providing value; from individual accountability to accountability at the organizational, professional, and industry levels; from defining and measuring quality to public transparency; from health services delivery to the domains of public health and health professionals' education. The research agenda has expanded from an academic specialty area to an imperative on which policy decisions are based.

Despite this progress, I still hear comments from students like "I wish my organization would operate that way," or "I wish my manager would learn this." The third edition of *Applying Quality Management to Healthcare* continues to aim to assist managers who are or will be operating in various levels and types of health services organizations rather than provide a comprehensive review of technical, medical, and policy issues related to quality of clinical care. The book is designed to enhance managers' literacy and awareness of concepts, topics, and practices required for effectively managing health services organizations in today's changing environment.

I use the term "manager" broadly. A "manager" is defined as "one that manages." The term "manage" is defined as "to exercise executive, administrative, and supervisory direction of" and "to succeed in accomplishing...to achieve one's purpose" (Merriam-Webster Online Dictionary 2010b). When the first definition is applied to quality, one considers the formal role of managers within an organization. Applying the second definition expands the application to programs, initiatives, and projects. Within this combined definition of the term "manage" this text approaches quality management. Quality management, in this text, refers to how managers operating in various types of health services organizations and settings understand, explain, and continuously improve their organizations to allow them to deliver quality and safe patient care, promote quality patient and organizational outcomes, and improve health in their communities.

This broader definition of "manage" and the focus of this text on improving understanding from a systems perspective have been well received by professionals in a wide range of health services settings. Students using the text have included those who manage hospitals, departments, and services (an oncology specialty hospital, inpatient care units, pharmacy services); manage professional practices (for physicians and nurse practitioners); manage agencies (public health and not-for-profit organizations); manage health programs (prevention, chronic disease, and children with special needs programs); manage a clinical service (pain); manage an academic department or division (pediatrics, surgery, obstetrics); and manage research projects (drug trials). Students have included physicians, nurses, pharmacists, educators, public health practitioners, and professionals with clinical and non-clinical backgrounds. One student, taking the quality management course as an elective for an MBA program, owned his own real estate business. The lessons gained prompted him to completely change his business model and approach.

The book strives to provide variety in its examples, though many are derived from clinical care. Readers are encouraged to consider the principles illustrated in the examples in relation to their own professional and work context and not just to the literal interpretation of the example. Just as in other domains of managerial knowledge, the principles and tools presented in this book may be widely applicable to a variety of settings.

The concepts and tools examined in this book come from varied disciplines, yet each has its origins in the systems perspective. When used together, their synergy provides managers with a guide to leveraging performance improvement and change efforts. In the past, quality management in healthcare has focused on tools to enhance a manager's ability to improve "how things are done" (process) and to "do the right things" (content). Increasingly, managers are also required to employ tools that examine underlying thinking and assumptions. To succeed in an uncertain environment, managers must know when to accept and when to challenge underlying assumptions.

The ability to understand and fluidly manage the relationship between traditional quality tools and tools that provide a deeper understanding of assumptions and other underlying systemic structures permits managers to continually raise the quality-management bar.

Changes from the Second Edition

As adoption of quality philosophies and approaches throughout the health services industry has grown, so has the availability of quality improvement and patient safety tools and resources. In response, this third edition provides a stronger emphasis on systems and a lesser emphasis on traditional quality tools and techniques. Chapter content continues to present concepts supported by real-life examples and illustrations.

Section I provides foundational content about systems and systems thinking. The Section I end-of-chapter exercises are designed to help students remember and understand systems concepts (Holt and Kysilka 2006).

Section II focuses on achieving results in complex systems and is generally organized according to the categories in the Baldrige Performance Excellence Program, Health Care Criteria for Performance Excellence: leadership (Chapter 5 "Establishing System Direction"); strategic planning (Chapter 6 "Establishing Improvement Goals in Complex Systems"); customer focus (Chapter 7 "Understanding Customer and Stakeholder Requirements"); organizational profile (Chapter 8 "Understanding the Role of Policy in Promoting System Change"); process management (Chapter 9 "Improving Processes and Implementing Improvements"); measurement, analysis, and knowledge management (Chapter 10 "Measuring Process and System Performance"); and workforce focus (Chapter 11 "Fostering Teamwork: Below-the-Waterline Considerations"). This section provides managers with frameworks, approaches, and tools to foster critical thinking by enhancing their ability to (Critical Thinking Community 2010)

- raise vital questions and problems, and formulate them clearly and precisely;
- gather and assess relevant information, use abstract ideas to interpret it effectively, come to well-reasoned conclusions and solutions, and test those conclusions against relevant criteria and standards;
- think open-mindedly within alternative systems of thought, and recognize and assess, as need be, assumptions, implications, and practical consequences; and
- communicate effectively with others to figure out solutions to complex problems.

The Section II end-of-chapter exercises are designed to promote the understanding and application of the content.

Section III represents an expanded version of the second edition epilogue using case studies and additional exercises designed for students to further apply, evaluate, and synthesize the content. These exercises are designed for students to individualize application to their own practice setting.

A glossary of terms has been added for quick reference, and each of the terms is also pulled out as a sidebar and defined within the chapter in which it appears.

Resources

Because of the rapidly changing environment relative to quality in the health services industry, the structure of the text has been designed to remain current while the third edition is in print. Selected companion readings supplement the text with more in-depth technical content and extend the application of chapter concepts with relevant and current issues faced by health services managers and leaders and provide readers with lists of leading authors and resources that may be followed for ongoing, up-to-date information. To support the teaching of this text, links to companion readings and Internet sites, explanations of exercises, and PowerPoint® slides are provided in an online Instructor Resource. For more information about the online Instructor Resources, please e-mail hap1@ache.org.

For students, end-of-chapter exercises, practice exercises, and web resources are available on this book's companion website at www.ache.org/books/qualitymanagement3.

ACKNOWLEDGMENTS

I extend my sincere gratitude to the individuals, students, teams, and organizations from whom and with whom I have learned over the years. Although impossible to list all of you by name, please know it is my privilege to call you colleagues. Knowing you and working with you has been crucial to the collective lessons presented in the book.

I am grateful to the many students who have provided feedback about the first two editions of the text and who have expanded my perspective. Many thanks to my editor, Eileen Lynch, and the rest of the wonderful staff at Health Administration Press for their hard work, collaboration, encouragement, and guidance.

Finally, I am indebted to my mentor, Dr. Arnold Kaluzny, whose continued support and belief in me made this book possible.

QUALITY MANAGEMENT: A SYSTEMS APPROACH

FUNDAMENTALS OF QUALITY MANAGEMENT

Learning Objectives

After completing this chapter you should be able to:

- describe the vital role of management to quality patient and client outcomes in health services organizations;
- define commonly used quality terms;
- differentiate between common approaches used to improve product and service quality;
- explain the three principles of total quality; and
- compare practices and traits as organizations mature along the quality continuum.

A mother arrives at the pediatrician's office for her daughter's six-month well-child checkup. As she has for previous checkups, she arrives ten minutes early and asks to occupy the well-child waiting area so her daughter will not pick up an infection from sick children in the regular waiting area. The scheduled appointment time of 10:00 am passes, and so do 10:30, 11:00, and 11:30. The nurse politely tells the mother that the pediatrician has been called to an emergency, saying, "I'm sure you understand. If it was your child, you would want the doctor to attend to her." Although the mother understands the reason for the delay, this explanation does not help the fact that she has to pick up her son from preschool at noon. The mother hunts for the harried nurse, who grabs a bite of her lunch each time she passes the nurse's station, to ask if her daughter may receive the required immunization shots and, if she could, to reschedule the rest of the checkup for another time.

Dissatisfied with the hours wasted at the pediatrician's office and disappointed with the need to return to finish the checkup, the mother demands to know if the pediatrician will be on emergency call during the time of the rescheduled appointment. When the mother and daughter arrive for the follow-up appointment, the mother hovers over the receptionist's desk so all of the staff will know she is ready and waiting. The office staff quickly identify this mother as a "problem."

While the pediatrician may possess a high level of clinical knowledge and competence, the mother's perception of her care is influenced by other factors, many of which fall within the domain of this pediatric office practice as a business. Regardless of the characteristics that define the pediatrician's business, the pediatrician is providing care within an organizational setting. In the broadest definition, an **organization** is a "social structure created by individuals to support the collaborative pursuit of specified goals" (Scott 2003, 11). In this example, the care providers and office staff are working together in the pursuit of children's healthcare services.

Organization
"social structure created by individuals to support the collaborative pursuit of specified goals" (Scott 2003, 11)

Why Focus on Management?

Viewing the pediatric practice as an "organization" implies that the pediatrician's clinical services are complemented with defined organizational functions. A deeper investigation of the design and execution of these functions provides clues to the mother's unsatisfactory experience. What are the specific goals of the practice and how are they determined? Does everyone in the practice understand and agree with these goals? How are patient appointments, office workflow, and staff hours scheduled to enable the practice to meet these goals? How are patient and family needs and expectations taken into account? Did the mother choose this pediatrician or was this the only one available based on her insurance plan? How are employees recruited, hired, trained, and evaluated? Does the pediatrician devote all of her time to the office or does she also have hospital commitments? How are responsibilities defined, coordinated, and balanced? How is the pediatrician compensated for services? How does reimbursement influence how work is done in the office? Does the practice operate according to a budget? Does the practice employ an office manager? If so, how is the manager's role defined? How do the pediatrician and the staff communicate with each other and with patients and their families?

Each of these questions represents a managerial choice about how the organization operates. Whether the organization purposefully chooses how it answers the previous questions or the questions are answered unknowingly by habit, default, or because "that's how we have always done it," the organizational functions represented by the questions still take place. In the example, the mother's experience resulted from how her pediatrician's practice did or did not address such questions. This mother's perception of quality had nothing to do with the quality of the *medical* care; it had everything to do with the quality of the *patient's* care.

The movement toward evidence-based medicine has resulted in numerous clinical guidelines representing best clinical practice. As illustrated in the example, in the absence of best organizational practice, patients may or may not receive the benefits of best clinical practice. This premise guides the focus of this text on management, because all health-related services are provided within and between *organizations.*

Although providing the service (e.g., performing cardiac surgery) and producing the product (e.g., ensuring clean water) are the functions of the clinical and technical professionals, the organizational functions described are the functions of management. A health services organization's methods of operation and organizational characteristics may differ according to its purpose, focus, and values. For example, the purpose of a health services organization may be care delivery, public health, education, or health promotion; the focus of a health services organization may be primary care, acute care, long-term care, or insurance and reimbursement; the operating values of a health services organization may be derived from its operating context such as urban or rural location, public or private ownership, or academic or community mission.

The manager's focus, perspective, and tactics may vary depending on his level (e.g., senior administrative, middle management, frontline supervisory) and his scope (e.g., team, project, department, division, agency, organization); however, all persons serving in a management role or holding management responsibilities in an organization are charged with finding ways to accomplish the aforementioned organizational functions.

Quality is not simply the responsibility of an organization's quality officer; patient safety is not simply the responsibility of the patient safety officer. Persons in these roles may be expert resources for providing information and helping managers understand, select, and implement tactics, interventions, and methods. The responsibility for ensuring quality and safe outcomes for patients, customers, stakeholders, and employees lies with those who determine how and what organizational objectives are set; how human, fiscal, material, and intellectual resources are secured, allocated, used, and preserved; and how activities in the organization are designed, carried out, coordinated, and improved.

The task of achieving quality outcomes from health services organizations is quickly becoming the shared responsibility of clinical professionals and management professionals. As Griffith and White (2005, 188) state, "just as medicine now follows guidelines for care; successful managers will use evidence and carefully developed processes to guide their decision making." The material presented in this book is intended to provide managers with evidence to assist them in improving their decision-making processes as they relate to quality and safety in their health services organizations.

What Is Quality?

The healthcare researcher's perspective may dominate definitions and approaches to quality in many settings. A widely accepted definition of **quality** as given by the Institute of Medicine is this: "The degree to which health services for individuals and populations increase the likelihood of desired

Quality
"The degree to which health services for individuals and populations increase the likelihood of desired health outcomes and are consistent with current professional knowledge" (Lohr 1990, 21)

Patient safety
"freedom from accidental or preventable injuries produced by medical care" (AHRQ 2010b)

health outcomes and are consistent with current professional knowledge" (Lohr 1990, 21). The corollary to quality is **patient safety**, defined as the "freedom from accidental or preventable injuries produced by medical care" (AHRQ 2010b).

The way practicing managers in health services organizations define and approach quality in the context of their daily responsibilities, however, may be influenced more by their own background and experiences. For example, a physician manager may emphasize clinical outcomes and the implementation of evidence-based medicine or clinical practice guidelines. A nurse manager may emphasize interpersonal skills, teamwork, and patient education. A public health specialist may emphasize disease management programs. Likewise, a non-clinical manager's educational focus may influence her preferred definition and approaches to quality. A manager educated in a business school may emphasize strategy, whereas someone trained as an accountant may emphasize the bottom line. A manager with a health services administration background may emphasize organizational structures and relationships.

Process of care
"a set of activities that go on within and between practitioners and patients" (Donabedian 1980, 79, 81–83)

These examples illustrate the assortment of perspectives and preferences about health services quality and the numerous ways quality concerns may be expressed within healthcare organizations. The multifaceted nature of quality poses several additional questions for healthcare managers: What is quality in healthcare? Which approach is best? How are the approaches related?

Structure
"the relatively stable characteristics of the providers of care, of the tools and resources they have at their disposal, and of the physical and organizational settings in which they work" (Donabedian 1980, 79, 81–83)

Since the early 1970s, Avedis Donabedian's work has influenced the prevailing medical paradigm of defining and measuring quality. In his early writings, Donabedian (1980) introduced the two essential parts—the technical components and the interpersonal components—that comprise quality medical care. He also identified three ways to measure quality (structure, process, and outcome) and the relationships among them. Donabedian (1980, 79, 81–83) described the measures in the following way:

Outcome
"a change in a patient's current and future health status that can be attributed to antecedent healthcare" (Donabedian 1980, 79, 81–83)

> I have called the **"process" of care** . . . a set of activities that go on within and between practitioners and patients. . . . Elements of the process of care do not signify quality until their relationship to desirable health status has been established. By **"structure"** I mean the relatively stable characteristics of the providers of care, of the tools and resources they have at their disposal, and of the physical and organizational settings in which they work. . . . Structure, therefore, is relevant to quality in that it increases or decreases the probability of good performance. . . . I shall use **"outcome"** to mean a change in a patient's current and future health status that can be attributed to antecedent healthcare. The fundamental functional relationships among the three elements are shown schematically as follows: Structure → Process → Outcome.

For example, in a family medicine group practice, the number and credentials of physicians, nurse practitioners, physician's assistants, nurses, and office staff are considered structure measures. The percentage of elderly patients who appropriately receive an influenza vaccine is considered a process measure, and the percentage of elderly patients who are diagnosed and treated for influenza is considered an outcome measure for this practice. The staff in the office (structure) would influence the ability of the practice to appropriately identify patients for whom the vaccine is indicated and to correctly administer the vaccine (process), which in turn would influence the number of patients developing influenza (outcome). If a process measure has a demonstrated link to an outcome, the process measure may be used as a proxy measure for an outcome.

Creating a Shared Definition of "Quality"

The concept of quality is "complex and represents a synthesis of lessons, methods, and acquired knowledge from a range of disciplines" (Dalrymple and Drew 2000, 697). While a health services manager can easily become overwhelmed by the complexity and extensive range of views on this topic, the manager may also consider this array of perspectives a vast pool from which to draw quality knowledge, lessons, and methods.

As with management practices, the subject of quality in healthcare organizations has been the object of numerous trends, fads, and attempts at quick fixes. Because departments and professionals with "quality" responsibilities may change their job titles with the latest trend, managers must understand what is behind the label; in other words, they must understand the philosophy and actions used to promote quality in an organization. The first step for managers is to develop a common understanding of quality terminology. Definitions of frequently used terms to describe quality are provided here.

Quality control is *(QC)* "the operational techniques and activities used to fulfill requirements for quality" (ASQ 2011)

Quality Control. Mostly used in the manufacturing setting, **quality control** (QC) encompasses "the operational techniques and activities used to fulfill requirements for quality" (ASQ 2011). In health services, quality control activities usually refer to equipment maintenance and calibration such as with the laboratory, imaging machines, and sterilization procedures.

Quality assurance (QA) eliminating defective outputs

Quality Assurance. A **quality assurance** (QA) approach is focused on the outputs of a process. Products are inspected after they are produced and imperfect products are discarded. In some cases, the defect may not be readily noticeable and is replaced at a later time, for example, as with a new automobile warranty. In a service industry, like healthcare, defects refer to unsatisfactory or defective outputs from a received service. The quality of the service is inspected after it is received and if not acceptable, the customer may ask for the service to be repeated; for example, a retail pharmacy

Quality improvement (QI)
improving defective processes to improve the quality of the outputs

Six Sigma
a rigorous and disciplined improvement approach using defined tools, methods, and statistical analysis with the goal of driving defects to zero

Lean thinking
an improvement philosophy based on eliminating waste

Toyota Production System
common method of applying Lean thinking in health services developed at the Toyota Motor Company

Total quality (TQ)
"a philosophy or an approach to management that can be characterized by its principles, practices, and techniques. Its three principles are customer focus, continuous improvement, and teamwork . . . each

includes only half the number of tablets in a prescription refill, and when the customer discovers this, he asks for the refill to be corrected. Sometimes the service defect is not readily noticeable, as in the case of an object left in a patient after a surgical procedure. As the patient's condition deteriorates, tests are performed to identify causes of the defective output. The patient must return to surgery for the defect to be corrected.

Quality Improvement. A **quality improvement** (QI) approach, also referred to as continuous quality improvement (CQI), is focused on improving defective processes to improve the quality of the outputs (i.e., reduce the number of defective outputs). Preoperative checklists, sponge counts, and team briefings are examples of operating room process improvements designed to prevent defective outputs or surgical complications. By improving the processes that deliver the outputs, QI seeks to produce defect-free products or to provide high-quality services consistently and dependably each time the service is provided.

Six Sigma. Based on the philosophy "that views all work as processes that can be defined, measured, analyzed, improved and controlled"(Benbow and Kubiak 2005, 1–2), **Six Sigma** is a rigorous and disciplined approach using improvement tools, methods, and statistical analysis. The phrase "six sigma" is a statistical term referring to the goal of driving defects to zero. Six Sigma quality is considered 3.4 defects per million (ASQ 2010c). Although the technique originated in manufacturing, the use of Six Sigma is growing in the health services arena.

Lean Thinking. **Lean thinking**, which also originated in manufacturing, is a philosophy based on eliminating waste. Lean thinking tools focus on production systems, scheduling, and wait times. The TPS (**Toyota Production System**) is a common method of applying lean thinking in health services organizations.

Total Quality. Because the term **total quality** (TQ), also referred to as total quality management or TQM, is often used interchangeably with the terms "QI" and "CQI," students and managers may be easily confused by these two related but different concepts. The following definition clarifies the differences between TQ and CQI. Total quality is "a philosophy or an approach to management that can be characterized by its principles, practices, and techniques. Its three principles are customer focus, continuous improvement, and teamwork . . . each principle is implemented through a set of practices . . . the practices are, in turn, supported by a wide array of techniques (i.e., specific step-by-step methods intended to make the practices effective)" (Dean and Bowen 2000, 4–5).

From this definition, one can see that TQ and CQI are not the same; TQ is a strategic concept, whereas CQI is one of three principles that support a TQ strategy. Numerous practices and techniques are available for managers to use in implementing the principles of CQI on a tactical and an operational level.

	Total Quality Theory	Management Theory
Audience	Managers	Researchers
Focus	Improve performance	Understand organizations

Source: Data from Dean and Bowen (2000).

EXHIBIT 1.1
Differences Between Total Quality Theory and Management Theory

Organizational Effectiveness. Not only must managers understand the differences between TQ and CQI, they must also understand the differences between quality theory and management theory, summarized in Exhibit 1.1.

The overlap of these two schools of thought is referred to as **organizational effectiveness**, a theoretical base that bridges the research–practice gap. Organizational effectiveness helps managers better understand and explain the organization (management theory) and also to improve the organization (total quality theory) (Dean and Bowen 2000).

Quality Management. In this book, the term **quality management** refers to the manager's role and contribution to organizational effectiveness. The book draws from management theory, quality theory as applied to non-healthcare organizations, and quality theory as applied to healthcare organizations to present practical lessons for managers and to integrate the unique characteristics of healthcare delivery and the context in which health services organizations operate. Quality management, for our purposes, refers to how managers operating in various types of health services organizations and settings understand, explain, and continuously improve their organizations to allow them to deliver quality and safe patient care, promote quality patient and organizational outcomes, and improve health in their communities.

Exhibit 1.2 provides a summary of the terms in this section and the actions these concepts require of the healthcare manager.

Three Principles of Total Quality

While the topics of customers, teams, and continuous improvement techniques are explored in depth in later chapters, a brief introduction to the three principles of total quality is provided in this section.

Customer Focus. A **customer** is defined as a user (or potential user) of one's services or programs (National Institute of Standards and Technology 2011). **External customers** are the parties outside the organization, and the primary external customers for health services providers are patients, families and significant others, clients, and communities. An **internal customer** is a user within the organization. Internal customers have been described as "someone whose inbox is your outbox" (unknown source). For example, in a hospital, when patient care is handed off from one provider to another

principle is implemented through a set of practices . . . the practices are, in turn, supported by a wide array of techniques (i.e., specific step-by-step methods intended to make the practices effective)" (Dean and Bowen 2000, 4–5)

Organizational effectiveness
a theoretical base resulting from the overlap of quality and management schools of thought that helps managers to better understand and explain the organization (management theory) and also to improve the organization (total quality theory) (Dean and Bowen 2000)

Quality management
the manager's role and contribution to organizational

EXHIBIT 1.2
Creating
a Shared
Definition:
Summary

Term	Practical Definition
Quality control (QC)	Fulfill requirements
Quality assurance (QA)	Find and repair faulty products
Quality improvement (QI/CQI)	Find and repair faulty processes
Six Sigma	Aggressively repair processes to reduce defects to zero
Lean thinking	Eliminate waste
Total quality (TQ/TQM)	Manage differently
Organizational effectiveness	Understand and improve the system

Source: Kelly (2009b).

effectiveness;
how managers
operating in
various types of
health services
organizations and
settings under-
stand, explain,
and continuously
improve their
organizations to
allow them to
deliver quality
and safe patient
care, promote
quality patient
and organizational
outcomes, and
improve health in
their communities

Customer
user or potential
user of one's ser-
vices or programs

External customer
a user outside the
organization

Internal customer
a user within the
organization

---

at shift change, the incoming provider is considered the internal customer of the outgoing provider. Completing the requisite shift responsibilities in a timely manner, communicating relevant information, and leaving a tidy work space demonstrate one's recognition of coworkers as internal customers.

The contemporary view of quality management expands the concept of "customer" to include stakeholders and markets in which the organization operates. The term **"stakeholder"** is used to refer to "all groups that are or might be affected by an organization's services, actions or success" (National Institute of Standards and Technology 2011, 63). In healthcare organizations, stakeholders may include "insurers and other third party payers, employers, health care providers, patient advocacy groups, Departments of Health, staff, partners, governing boards, investors, charitable contributors, suppliers, taxpayers, policymakers, and local and professional communities" (National Institute of Standards and Technology 2011, 63). Defining customers and stakeholders is a prerequisite to determining their requirements and, in turn, to designing organizational processes that meet these requirements.

Continuous Improvement. When the manager of an environmental services department in a large hospital picks up something from the hallway floor and throws it away in the nearest trash can, her action exemplifies the principle of continuous improvement. While other hospital employees might walk past the trash, the environmental services manager realizes the importance of being committed to continuous improvement for her department and for the hospital; if at any time the manager sees something that needs fixing, improving, or correcting, she takes the initiative. If managers want to achieve continuous improvement in their organizations, they must demonstrate continuous improvement through their everyday actions.

The principle of continuous improvement may also be expressed through managers' execution of their managerial functions. Managing by fact and depending on performance data to inform decisions is requisite to this principle. Depending on the nature of the work and the scope of management responsibility, performance data may be reported at various time intervals. For example, a shift supervisor for the patient transportation service in an 800-bed academic medical center watches the electronic dispatch system that displays a minute-by-minute update on transportation requests, indicators of patients en route to their destination, and the number of patients in the queue. By monitoring the system, the supervisor is immediately aware if a problem occurs and, as a result, is able to take action quickly to resolve the problem. If the number of requests unexpectedly increases, the supervisor can reassign staff breaks to maximize staff availability and minimize response times.

Each day, the supervisor posts the total number of transports performed the previous day along with the average response times. This way, the patient transporters are aware of the department's statistics and their own individual statistics, and this helps the transporters take pride in a job that is typically underappreciated by others in the organization. The daily performance data also enable the supervisor to quickly identify documented complaints and to address them within 24 hours, which in turn increases employee accountability and improves customer relations. On a monthly basis, the department manager and the shift supervisors review the volume of requests by hour of the day to determine if employees are scheduled appropriately to meet demand. The manager also reviews the statistics sorted by patient unit (e.g., nursing unit, radiology department) to identify any issues that need to be explored directly, manager to manager. The manager reviews the monthly statistics with his administrator, and the annual statistics are used in the budgeting process.

A performance measurement and management system such as this enables managers to continually monitor performance; to identify quality issues and performance gaps and to take action to resolve them; and to provide a foundation for ongoing communication, planning, and accountability.

Teamwork. In many organizations, when the terms "teamwork" and "quality" are used together, they usually refer to cross-functional or interdisciplinary project teams. In relation to quality management, managers should also consider teamwork when they carry out functions inherent in the managerial role, in particular, organizational design, resource allocation, and communication.

Organizational design has been identified as a critical management function and encompasses "how the building blocks of the organization (authority, responsibility, accountability, information, and rewards) are arranged and rearranged to improve effectiveness and adaptive capacity" (Shortell and Kaluzny 2006, 316). The principle of teamwork implies that managers proactively and purposefully arrange the organization's building blocks at all levels—for individual positions and work groups and at departmental and organizational levels—in a manner that supports teamwork.

Stakeholder
"all groups that are or might be affected by an organization's services, actions or success" (National Institute of Standards and Technology 2011, 63)

Organizational design
"how the building blocks of the organization (authority, responsibility, accountability, information, and rewards) are arranged and rearranged to improve effectiveness and adaptive capacity" (Shortell and Kaluzny 2006, 316)

Some organizational designs, such as a matrix structure or a service-line structure, may promote teamwork. A matrix structure is characterized by a dual-authority system. In a service-line structure, a single person is responsible for all aspects of a group of services, usually based on patient type (e.g., pediatric, women's services, oncology, transplant services) (Shortell and Kaluzny 2006).

One large hospital used a hybrid of these two structures in its approach to organizational design. Each administrator was responsible for multiple departments that cared for patients with similar needs. For example, the trauma administrator was responsible for the emergency department, the trauma intensive care unit, and the air transport service. Although finance, human resources, and quality resources operated from their own centralized departments to maintain their unique competencies, each administrator in the hospital was assigned finance, human resources, and quality "consultants." Teamwork between the administrators and the dedicated staff consultants enhanced the staff's ability to provide consistent and responsive service to the administrators and the managers for whom they were responsible.

Promoting effective interdependence between care team members implies the need for trust and understanding among team members. Building working relationships is difficult in environments that experience high turnover or that are staffed with continuous streams of temporary employees. While in the past activities such as recruitment and retention might have fallen under the responsibilities of the human resources department, managers today must be keenly aware of the way human resources issues affect their ability not only to fulfill the quality management principle of teamwork but also to promote quality patient outcomes and cost effectiveness.

Designing and implementing decision-making, documentation, and communication processes (which ensure individuals and teams have the information they need, when they need it, to make effective and timely clinical and organizational decisions) reflect a manager's understanding of the quality management principles. For example, in one hospital, the manager of the materials management department negotiates with a supplier to obtain surgical gloves at a discounted rate compared to the rate of the current supplier; the decision is made based on vendor and financial input. The first time the new gloves are used, however, the surgeon rips out the fingers of the gloves while inserting his hand. Had the manager embraced the concept of teamwork in her approach to decision making, she would have sought out information and input from the patient care team—the people who actually use the product and know the advantages and disadvantages of different brands of gloves.

Quality Continuum for Managers

Quality management is not a single event; rather, it is a journey. Progress along the journey may be viewed on a continuum with one end representing traditional or early attempts at quality and the other end representing more mature approaches (Exhibit 1.3). The first decade of the twenty-first century witnessed the increasing use of regulatory requirements, accreditation standards, transparency, and consumer activism to speed the movement of health services organizations along the quality continuum. These initiatives will be described in more detail in Chapter 8.

In the United States, The Joint Commission is one accrediting body for health services organizations. Readers who began their professional roles after The Joint Commission implemented its redesigned accreditation process in 2004 may not be familiar with the "old" approach to preparing for a hospital accreditation survey. As of 2004, The Joint Commission "focuses on improving the safety and quality of care provided through continuous standards compliance" (The Joint Commission 2005), an approach representing the mature end of the quality continuum. Comparing this new philosophy with the traditional philosophy of preparing for a hospital accreditation survey illustrates the quality continuum.

Hospital A is a large academic medical center. More than 15 years ago, its chief executive officer (CEO) demonstrated his support for quality by changing the QA department to the CQI department and hiring a director of CQI. The department organizational chart consists of the accreditation coordinator and the CQI coordinator who both report to the CQI director. The accreditation coordinator supervises three staff members; they are responsible for hospital accreditation preparation and for collecting and reporting the performance measures required by The Joint Commission. The CQI coordinator supervises five staff members; they assist teams throughout the hospital with improvement projects by providing facilitation, teaching improvement tools, and collecting and reporting data on the improvements.

Hospital A goes through The Joint Commission accreditation survey every three years, and the survey preparation process has been the same for as long as anyone can remember. Nine months before the review, the accreditation coordinator develops a master task list. The coordinator and his staff meet with every department manager to give out assignments and the timeline for completion. At the monthly hospital managers' meeting, the coordinator provides a progress report and announces the "countdown until the accreditation survey." Three months before the survey, the coordinator's staff works six days a week. The last month before the review, the CQI staff work 12 hours a day, six days a week. The level of stress in the organization gradually increases over the nine months of preparation, and the organization is in a state of frenzy a few weeks before the review. The surveyors arrive. The review is successfully completed, and the hospital even receives high praise for two of the CQI presentations the CQI coordinator prepared.

Hospital B is also a large academic medical center. Until ten years ago, the hospital approached The Joint Commission review process in a manner similar to that of Hospital A. At that time, a new CEO was hired, and as she was getting acquainted with managers throughout the hospital, she asked a simple question: "What would happen if we operated every day as if The Joint Commission were coming?" Systematically, she began to create an organizational culture that she believed would be the answer to her question.

Hospital B also had two separate quality-department groups: one group was focused on accreditation and one group was involved in facilitating CQI projects. The first thing the new CEO did was to merge the two groups into one and rename the department as the quality resources department. Rather than make the quality resources department the entity solely responsible for quality-related activities in the hospital, the CEO redefined the role of every manager throughout the hospital to include expectations for performance results, improvement projects, and accreditation. Each manager was assigned a dedicated quality consultant from the quality resources department who would serve as a resource on measurement; data collection and analysis; The Joint Commission standards; and improvement tools, methods, and facilitation. Some quality consultants supported many small units, and some quality consultants supported a few large units.

The CEO also set new expectations for the administrators who reported to her. With her administrative team, she began to review monthly reports on patient satisfaction, financial performance, clinical outcomes, and productivity. As a group, they reviewed trends and discussed performance-related issues. After a year, the CEO asked the administrators to set their own performance goals based on opportunities identified from these monthly performance discussions. In turn, the administrators worked with the managers who reported to them to set department-level goals that were consistent with the administrative-level performance goals. All department managers were involved. For example, the pharmacy manager set the goal to improve the time to fill an outpatient prescription, and the finance manager set the goal to design financial reports that were more useful to managers.

The CEO also redesigned the hospital newsletter to include a "CEO Update" column that reported the hospital's performance and any business or market issues affecting the hospital. Finally, the CEO dug out employee satisfaction survey results from the past several years. She studied them as part of setting her own goals to address sources of employee dissatisfaction. She considered the responsibility of creating the culture and providing the environment, resources, and tools that would best enable employees to deliver quality care to patients to be her responsibility.

As The Joint Commission review date approaches for Hospital B, announcements are made and final details are addressed. The week of the surveyors' visit is seen as "business as usual." The survey is successfully completed without much stress.

Hospital A exemplifies a traditional or less mature approach to quality. The focus is on meeting standards and eliminating defects. Quality is the job of specialists, while responsibilities for accreditation and continuous improvement belong to the CQI department. The hospital takes small steps along the continuum when it adopts CQI techniques to improve work processes.

Hospital B exemplifies an organization that is progressing to a more mature state along the quality continuum. Hospital leaders demonstrate quality through their actions and through the direction they set for the organization. Quality is the responsibility of everyone in the organization rather than something delegated to specialists. Requirements of internal and external customers and stakeholders are recognized and addressed. All processes in the organization—clinical patient-care processes and internal operational and administrative processes—are targeted for improvement. Ongoing measurement and feedback promote an understanding of past and current performance to support the organization's ability to continually improve its results for patients and other stakeholders.

Although a healthcare organization may occupy a point anywhere along this maturity continuum, the goal of quality management is to continually strive toward the most mature end of the continuum. Exhibit 1.3 illustrates how the continuum may be viewed for healthcare organizations.

An understanding of the quality continuum in health services organizations begins to explain differences in operations and outcomes in organizations that all claim to be "quality organizations," such as

- how an organization can be successful at quality projects but not attain a quality organizational culture;
- why some organizations have adjusted better than others to the current process for accreditation;
- why defining clinical practice guidelines does not in itself guarantee healthcare quality;
- why organizational development efforts, independent of clinical context, may not yield expected results; and
- why, without leadership's involvement in establishing a quality philosophy and strategy for the entire organization, only pockets of excellence may be found in an organization.

Summary

The information presented in this text is not intended to replace management knowledge and skills in areas such as finance, human resources, strategy, or marketing; rather, this information should complement those areas. This chapter has introduced various terms and approaches to aid managers in establishing a common definition of quality in their organizations. The path to becoming a mature quality organization is a process characterized by transitions in managerial philosophy, thinking, and action.

EXHIBIT 1.3
Quality
Continuum
for Healthcare
Managers

- Meet standards
- Eliminate defects

- Products:
  Healthcare delivery

- Processes: Clinical
  procedures/support
  processes
- Customers: Patients,
  physicians
- Clients who buy the
  products: Patients,
  payers

- Cost of poor quality:
  Financial

- Products: All products,
  goods, and services, whether
  for sale or not—care delivery,
  public healthcare, payers,
  equipment, supplies
- Processes: All processes—
  clinical, business, operational,
  support, manufacturing,
  decision making, policy
- Customers and other stakeholders: Anyone who has an
  expectation of, is interested in,
  or is affected by the work of
  the organization—patients,
  families, internal customers,
  employers, communities,
  organizations, regulators
- Costs of poor quality:
  All costs that would disappear
  if everything were perfect—
  financial, quality-of-life,
  productivity, and opportunity
  costs

Less Mature ——————————————————————→ **More Mature**

Source: Adapted with the permission of The Free Press, a Division of Simon & Schuster Adult Publishing Group, from *Juran on Leadership for Quality: An Executive Handbook* by J. M. Juran (p. 48). Copyright © 1989 by Juran Institute, Inc. All rights reserved.

Exercise I

Background: In 2001, the Institute of Medicine published *Envisioning the National Health Care Quality Report*, which recommended the development of a report that "should serve as a yardstick or barometer by which to gauge progress in improving the performance of the health care delivery system in consistently providing high-quality care." In 2003, the Agency for Healthcare Research and Quality published the first annual National Healthcare Quality Report along with its companion National Healthcare Disparities Report.

Objective: To explore the current state of healthcare quality in the United States.

Instructions:
- Go to the AHRQ website (www.ahrq.gov) and find the most current versions of these two reports.
- Read the Key Themes and Highlights sections.

- Browse the rest of the report.
- Based on your brief review of these two reports, write a one-paragraph summary of the state of healthcare quality in the United States.

Exercise II

Background: The Kaiser Family Foundation (KFF) is a private, not-for-profit foundation devoted to healthcare and health policy issues. One section of its website is called the United States Global Health Policy section. This section collects and presents health data from numerous sources in a user-friendly format.

Objective: To explore the current state of health in the United States.

Instructions:
- Go to the Country Data section of the KFF United States Global Health Policy website: www.globalhealthfacts.org
- Find the following population health and financial indicators: infant mortality rate, male and female life expectancy, obesity and smoking prevalence, total health expenditures, and government health expenditure as percent of total government.
- Review and compare the US data with that of other developed countries.
- Based on your brief review of these data, write a one-paragraph summary of the state of health in the United States compared to other developed countries.

Web Resources

Agency for Healthcare Research and Quality: www.ahrq.gov
American Society for Quality: www.asq.org/
National Association for Healthcare Quality: www.nahq.org/

Companion Readings

Goldhill, D. 2009. "How American Health Care Killed My Father." *Atlantic Monthly* 304 (2): 38–55.

Griffith, J. R., and K. R. White. 2005. "The Revolution in Hospital Management." *Journal of Healthcare Management* 50 (3): 170–90.

Institute of Medicine. 2001. *Crossing the Quality Chasm: A New Health System for the 21st Century.* [Online publication; released 3/1/01.] www.iom.edu/Reports/2001/Crossing-the-Quality-Chasm-A-New-Health-System-for-the-21st-Century.aspx

———. 1999. *To Err Is Human: Building a Safer Health System.* [Online publication; released 11/1/99.] www.iom.edu/Reports/1999/To-Err-is-Human-Building-A-Safer-Health-System.aspx

A SYSTEMS PERSPECTIVE OF QUALITY MANAGEMENT: CHARACTERISTICS OF COMPLEX SYSTEMS

Learning Objectives

After completing this chapter you should be able to:

- discuss how a systems perspective can explain recurrent organizational problems;
- define the terms "system," "systems thinking," and "dynamic complexity";
- describe system characteristics that contribute to dynamic complexity;
- identify the influence of dynamic complexity on health services organizations; and
- understand the implications of dynamic complexity on managerial decision making.

As people accumulate years of experience in the healthcare field, they begin to see the recurring problems—sometimes within an individual organization, sometimes across the entire industry. Problems thought to be solved by one manager may come back at a later time for a different manager. The vice president of nursing of a large hospital may centralize and cross-train nurse educator positions to meet necessary budget cuts for the year; three years later, the new vice president of nursing of the same hospital adds unit-based nurse educator positions to address unmet clinical orientation needs of its new hires. Consider the following situation (Georgopoulos and Mann 1962, 549–51):

> The hospital faces a number of problems concerning the nursing staff . . . one major problem is . . . attracting and retaining a sufficient professional nursing staff, especially non-supervisory nursing staff. . . . [T]he problem lies in the fact that the number of professional nurses being trained in nursing schools is much too low to meet an ever increasing demand for professional nurses by hospitals and other sources. . . . [B]eing understaffed, hospitals often assign to the professional nurse a rather heavy workload that is not seen

as normal or reasonable by many nurses. . . . [A]nother important problem . . . involves the composition of the total nursing staff, the question of optimum balance in the proportions of staff members who are registered nurses, practical nurses, and aides.

Although this situation may appear to address a manager's current challenges with nursing shortages, the excerpt was taken from the book *The Community General Hospital*, which was published in 1962! During the 60 years since that book was written, health services organizations seem to have made little headway in issues related to workforce planning and management. Nursing shortages, for example, appeared and disappeared in waves in the 1960s, 1970s, 1980s, early 1990s, and again in the early decades of the twenty-first century. Compounding the current nursing shortage is a nursing faculty shortage: "US nursing schools turned away 54,991 qualified applicants from baccalaureate and graduate nursing programs in 2009 due to an insufficient number of faculty" (AACN 2010).

Why do budget problems and workforce shortages remain nagging issues for health services managers? The reasons lie in the complex nature of healthcare, healthcare organizations, and the healthcare industry. In healthcare, as in other industries, "systems thinking is needed more than ever because we are being overwhelmed with complexity" (Senge 1990, 69). Today, one may rephrase Senge's 1990 comment to read, "systems thinking is imperative in health services organizations because they are much more complex than they were in 1990."

Returning to the hospital staffing example, one begins to see how the complexity of professional, financial, and operational drivers of human resources allocation today has increased over time. One example is the impact of generational differences in the workplace. The four generations are referred to as traditionalists or veterans (born 1922–1946), baby boomers (born 1946–1964), generation X (born 1964–1980), and millenials (born 1980–2000) (Houlihan 2007). In health services organizations, generational differences influence the caregiver and the care recipient, and a mismatch between the caregiver's generational communication preferences and care receiver's generational communication preferences can affect the patient's experience and outcomes of care. For example, one manager sought to better understand the influence of generational differences on patient satisfaction in her labor and delivery unit. When the potential combinations of patients and the nurses caring for them were mapped according to their generations (shown in Exhibit 2.1), the complexity of her "simple" question became immediately apparent (Gulliver and Kelly 2009).

Other variables influencing hospital staffing include an aging workforce; the growing proportion of the US elderly population with their accompanying chronic illnesses; cultural diversity and language differences of workers and patients; prevalence of hospitalized patients suffering from morbid

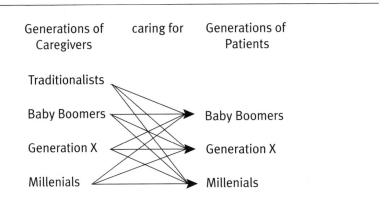

EXHIBIT 2.1
Generational
Combinations
Between
Patients and
Caregivers

obesity; clinical and information technology; and emerging infectious diseases such as Methicillin-resistant *Staphylococcus aureus* (MRSA) and H1N1.

When speaking about systems, the term **complex** refers to the presence of a large number of variables that interact with each other in countless and often unpredictable ways. A quick exploration of the generational issue reveals that a single nurse-to-patient relationship expanded to 12 possibilities of generational combinations. This example represents one nurse on one shift with one patient on one unit. Considering the multiple determinants of health and the vast number of components that comprise health services organizations, the possibilities of interaction are mind-boggling. Health and health services organizations are also characterized by situations in which "cause and effect are subtle, and where the effects over time of interventions are not obvious" (Senge 2006, 71). This characteristic represents another type of complexity, known as **dynamic complexity**. In the presence of dynamic complexity, "the same action has dramatically different effects in the short run and the long run . . . an action has one set of consequences locally and a very different set of consequences in another part of the system . . . and obvious interventions produce nonobvious consequences" (Senge 2006, 71). When faced with dynamic complexity, managers must select interventions that alter the fundamental behavior of the system that is causing the problem; otherwise the solution is only temporary. As seen in the nursing shortage example, although interventions may offer temporary relief, the problems resurface again and again.

This chapter introduces a systems perspective of quality management that is based on the concepts of systems thinking and dynamic complexity.

Complex
the presence of a large number of variables that interact with each other in innumerable ways

Dynamic complexity
where "cause and effect are subtle, and where the effects over time of interventions are not obvious" (Senge 2006, 71)

Systems Thinking

In Chapter 1, a variety of perspectives surrounding the term "quality" are discussed. Likewise, the term "system" brings with it numerous connotations and perceptions. While "system change" is often heard in the quality and safety discourse, the term "system" may be defined and perceived in a variety of ways. In this book, a **system** refers to a collection of parts that interact with each other to form an interdependent whole (Kauffman 1980; Scott 2003).

A system reflects the whole, and "**systems thinking** is a discipline for seeing wholes. It is a framework for seeing interrelationships, rather than things; for seeing patterns of change rather than static 'snap-shots' . . . and systems thinking is a sensibility—for the subtle interconnectedness that gives living systems their unique character" (Senge 2006, 68–69). Systems thinking acknowledges the large number of parts in a system, the infinite number of ways in which the parts interact, and the nature of the interactions. Systems thinking requires that one look for relationships between the elements of a system and seek to understand how they are connected.

Dynamic Complexity

Several system characteristics contribute to the presence of dynamic complexity (Sterman 2000). Five characteristics, predominant in healthcare and health services organizations, are described in this section: change, trade-offs, history dependency, tight coupling, and nonlinearity.

Change

Systems are dynamic—that is, changing. Change occurs at different rates and scales within and among systems, especially in healthcare. Consider three levels of this characteristic of dynamic complexity in health services. First, the human body changes continuously. This means that key inputs (patients with a clinical problem) to and outputs (patients' status after clinical intervention) of healthcare systems are moving targets. Second, the organizational contexts in which health services are carried out are dynamic in nature. Employees move in and out of organizations, research provides an ongoing stream of new evidence, and technological advances offer new clinical and management approaches. Third, the communities and political environments in which we live and in which healthcare organizations operate change—that is, the environment changes with economic cycles, political ideologies, and election cycles.

From the day a person is born to the day she dies, she is in a constant state of change, growing and developing physiologically and emotionally. No two human systems are alike or precisely predictable in their response to a medical intervention. As a result, functions that may seem straightforward in other industries, such as product standardization, become more difficult for healthcare managers. For example, the practice of using a standardized list of drug names and brands (i.e., a hospital formulary) to reduce medication expenses is accepted practice. However, when the dynamic nature of patient physiology is introduced, the manager recognizes that in addition to the question, "What are the set of drug names and brands that will be most cost-effective?" he also needs to ask, "How should the approved drugs be selected, and what are the consequences to patients?"

To aid in grasping the subtle but important nuances involved in individualizing treatment plans, the metaphor of trying on a pair of blue jeans may be used. People have their own favorite brand of blue jeans that "fit," even though another brand may be advertised as having a similar size and style. The formulary essentially dictates to doctors that the patient may buy only slim-cut size 10 jeans and not relaxed-fit size 10 jeans (Kelly and Pestotnik 1998). Research on variations in genetic makeup and the nature of gene–environment interactions promises to shed light in yet unimaginable ways on why certain treatments or medications may work better for one person than another. The emerging fields of **pharmacogenomics** may permit drug selection in the future to be based on an individual's unique genetic makeup, altering the paradigm on which health services organizations manage **pharmacotherapeutics**, "the study of the therapeutic uses and effects of drugs" (Medline Plus Merriam-Webster Medical Dictionary 2011). Preemptive medicine—"removing the initial molecular event—precluding the possibility of that thing even happening" (Culliton 2006, W96)—will likely alter the fundamental role of healthcare delivery organizations in the future.

Trade-Offs

The need to understand the nature of trade-offs may seem unnecessary for managers taught to weigh pros versus cons or opportunities versus risks as they consider organizational decision options. Trade-offs may be seen as an accepted attribute of management. However, an understanding of dynamic complexity fosters an appreciation for the system consequences of local management trade-off decisions. "Time delays in feedback channels mean the long-run response of a system to an intervention is often different from its short-run response. High leverage policies often cause worse-before-better behavior, while low leverage policies often generate transitory improvement before the problem grows worse" (Sterman 2000, 22).

A classic example of a low-leverage policy was published in the *New England Journal of Medicine* (Fitzgerald, Moore, and Dittus 1988). Although a 1988 publication may be viewed as dated, the lessons for managers in this article are more relevant today than when the study was published.

The advent of prospective payment systems in 1983 drove many hospitals to reduce costs by decreasing patient length of stay. This article examined the effect of these practices on quality of care for elderly patients with hip fractures. As Exhibit 2.2 summarizes, the variables studied included length of

---

Pharmacogenomics

"a science that examines the inherited variations in genes that dictate drug response and explores the ways these variations can be used to predict whether a patient will have a good response to a drug, a bad response to a drug, or no response at all" (NCBI 2004)

Pharmacotherapeutics

"the study of the therapeutic uses and effects of drugs" (Medline Plus Merriam-Webster Medical Dictionary 2011)

Implications for Healthcare Managers

EXHIBIT 2.2		**Before**	**After**
Impact of Low-Leverage Policy: Reducing Hospital Costs by Reducing Hospital Length of Stay	Length of stay	21.9 days	12.6 days
	Physical therapy sessions	7.6	6.3
	Functional status (measured by distance in feet walked)	93	38
	Percentage of patients discharged to nursing homes	38%	60%
	Percentage of patients still in nursing homes one year after discharge	9%	33%

Source: Adapted with permission from Table 2 in "The Care of Elderly Patients with Hip Fracture. Changes Since Implementation of the Prospective Payment System" by J. F. Fitzgerald, P. S. Moore, and R. S. Dittus, in the *New England Journal of Medicine* 319 (21): 1394. Copyright © 1988 Massachusetts Medical Society. All rights reserved.

stay, number of physical therapy sessions, functional status measured by the distance in feet that patients could walk, percentage of patients discharged to nursing homes, and percentage of patients still in nursing homes one year after discharge. If a manager in this case defined the healthcare system as "the orthopedic department/unit" or the hospital administrator defined the healthcare system as "this hospital," the intervention chosen to reduce healthcare system costs appeared to be appropriate. In this article, the decision and subsequent interventions to reduce hospital length of stay appeared to be successful; mean hospital stay declined from 21.9 to 12.6 days. In addition, "neither in-hospital mortality nor one-year mortality changed significantly" (Fitzgerald, Moore, and Dittus 1988, 1392). Based on these criteria—length of hospital stay, hospital mortality, and one-year mortality—a manager could be confident that this was a successful cost-reduction strategy.

However, if one defines the healthcare system as including not only the acute phase of care (e.g., orthopedic unit, hospital) but also the downstream providers (e.g., rehabilitation, long-term care) and takes into account how the relationships among all providers influence patient outcomes, the longer-term behavior of the system can be observed. The short-term intervention of reducing hospital length of stay and in turn reducing physical therapy sessions and functional status also led to an increase in patients discharged from the hospital directly to nursing homes. The authors concluded that the result was a shift in "much of the rehabilitation burden to nursing homes" (Fitzgerald, Moore, and Dittus 1988, 1392), and they observed a subsequent increase in the percentage of patients remaining in nursing homes one year after hospital discharge. Overall costs related to the consumption of healthcare resources for the care of these patients actually increased.

To this finding, a manager may respond, "But my responsibility is only my unit/hospital." From a systems perspective, the acute care manager is responsible not simply for the acute care unit or hospital but also for the effect those local decisions have on the rest of the system of which the manager's component is a part. This does not mean that the manager of the orthopedic department or the hospital administrator should not strive to reduce hospital costs. It does mean, however, that managers, financial officers, CEOs, and policymakers should be aware of how decisions made and implemented within their domains of responsibility affect other parts of the healthcare system, positively and negatively. When a negative impact to another part of the system is anticipated, the manager should be proactive in the short term to help minimize the negative effects and preserve positive patient outcomes. In the case presented in this article, a proactive intervention would have been to ensure that nursing homes had adequate rehabilitation capacity before reducing hospital length of stay. These challenges have been addressed over the years and are seen today in improvements to post-acute care, strengthened relationships between acute care and skilled nursing facilities (SNFs), and the emergence of the concept of **accountable care organizations** (ACOs).

Accountable care organization (ACO) an organization through which groups of providers share responsibility for providing care (Gold 2011)

Other common trade-off challenges for healthcare managers surround the differences between expense and investment decisions within organizations and departments. The long-term effect of a manager's short-term decision may not be felt by another component in the system (e.g., nursing home, patient) as in the previous example, but perhaps it will surface at a certain point in the future within the manager's own department or organization. For example, does the manager sacrifice capital improvements to fund agency workers in the short term? Do managers reduce staff education dollars to reduce current expenses? Although choosing agency workers and reducing staff development activities may meet the short-term need to reduce expenses, these efforts fall into the category of low-leverage policies because the problems of facility aging, staff shortages, and the need for a competent workforce will surely be faced by the manager in the future. Without an appreciation of system consequences, one manager may be rewarded for the short-term "success" with a promotion, while his successor inherits the longer-term problem.

In the formulary example, the organization may be willing to trade the rare adverse medication event for dollar savings realized from product standardization. However, this type of micro (patient level)/macro (organizational level) trade-off that allows for patient status to be potentially compromised may unintentionally contribute to polarization and conflict between clinicians and managers.

History Dependency

Systems are history dependent. In other words, what has happened in the past influences what is occurring in the present. Some actions are reversible, but many actions are not.

Implications for Healthcare Managers

History dependency may be seen in the patient and the organization. Due to advancements in care of chronic illnesses, rather than succumb to complications of one illness, elderly adults are often under treatment for several chronic illnesses concurrently. Persons with cystic fibrosis or born with congenital heart defects now enjoy a life expectancy into adulthood; previously these conditions usually were fatal in childhood. Unhealthy behaviors, such as excessive alcohol, drugs, or cigarettes, even when discontinued, may have long-lasting health consequences. Understanding a patient's history is not only important for clinical providers, but also is important for health services managers. For example, a patient's health history influences resources required for his care. An obese patient being treated for asthma, hypertension, and diabetes requires more labor-intensive care when having his gallbladder removed than an otherwise healthy athlete undergoing the same surgery. In recognition of these differences, clinical outcomes analysis requires adjustments for patient acuity (e.g., presence of comorbidities) and definition of an organization's overall patient acuity (e.g., case mix index [CMI]) (Iezzoni 2003). Such analytic tools take into account the patient as a dynamic system and permit comparison of outcomes between different patients and institutions.

Another example of this characteristic is how a healthcare organization's past decision to pursue or not pursue electronic information systems affects its ability to meet current information demands and reporting requirements. The ability of the healthcare industry to manage information and report performance pales in comparison to that of other industries, such as financial services. Consider the following perspective: "If you go to the doctor, the doctor is recording your visit in vegetable pigment on crushed wood fibers. This is literally a medieval method of data storage and retrieval. I ask you, how would you react if you went to a bank and asked for money and someone opened up a big, old ledger and blew it off and said, 'Oh, let's see, how much do you have?'" (Smith 2002).

The manager must realize not only how past events have shaped current events but also how past decision-making strategies and directions may influence her ability to successfully achieve current and future goals. Using the information systems example, if the organization has historically rewarded managers for quarterly or annual financial performance, a large capital investment today for a future financial gain may be difficult to sell given the reward and decision-making history of the organization.

Tight Coupling

A system is characterized as **tightly coupled** when "the parts exhibit relatively time-dependent, invariant, and inflexible connections with little slack" (Scott 2003, 358), as in elegantly crafted configurations of dominoes that are set in motion by a push to the first piece. Tight coupling is also present when "the actors in the system interact strongly with one another" (Sterman 2000, 22).

Tightly coupled when the parts of a system "exhibit relatively time-dependent, invariant, and inflexible connections with little slack" (Scott 2003, 358)

Implications for Healthcare Managers

Organizations in industries outside of health services that are most commonly identified as tightly coupled include nuclear power plants and aircraft carriers (Roberts 1990). Health services, however, are not contained within a single organization; rather, services are provided by a complex variety of interdependent organizations (i.e., social structures; see Chapter 1). Within these organizations, nested structures such as departments, divisions, and professional groups are also present. Social organizations are generally considered to be "complex and loosely coupled" (Scott 2003, 83); however, the tasks carried out by the organizations may often be considered tightly coupled. For example, surgeons, anesthesiologists, and nurses may belong to separate, distinct, loosely coupled departments within the structure of the organization, yet, when they come together in the operating suite, the tasks involved in conducting a surgical procedure are tightly coupled. An undetected mistaken patient identity or incorrect surgical site can quickly lead to disastrous consequences if not identified prior to surgery.

Tools such as the World Health Organization Surgical Safety Checklist are intended to align the loosely and tightly coupled parts of the system to promote safe clinical outcomes in any surgical setting with any team of providers. This tool specifies the items that must be verified and who must verify them prior to three key phases of the surgical procedure: at anesthesia induction, at incision, and when the patient leaves the operating room (WHO 2010). Likewise, immediately placing identification on newborns, especially with multiple births, is standard practice. Consider twins whose identification bands are accidentally switched at birth. The twins subsequently could receive multiple inappropriate treatment orders as all diagnostic results and other documentation are mistakenly applied to the wrong baby.

Numerous interactions within and between people, processes, and departments within individual organizations and interactions among services along the continuum of care require managers to be attentive to the concept of coupling. Identifying, designing, and institutionalizing tools that promote task alignment, communication, collaboration, coordination, and strengthened relationships among the players are required competencies for contemporary health services managers.

Nonlinear
the "effect is
rarely propor-
tional to the
cause" (Sterman
2000, 22)

Nonlinearity

The term **nonlinear**, as it refers to a system characteristic, means that the "effect is rarely proportional to the cause" (Sterman 2000, 22) and that, because the parts in the system may interact in numerous ways, these interactions may follow "unexpected sequences that are not visible or not immediately comprehensible" (Scott 2003, 358).

Implications for Healthcare Managers

A nurse just starting the afternoon shift is the object of an outburst of anger from a patient's family. The nurse relates the encounter to a colleague at the nurse's station: "All I did was say, 'Hello'!" This situation may bring to mind the old cliché "the straw that broke the camel's back." In fact, this cliché is an accurate description of the encounter.

The patient and her family had accumulated a sequence of unsatisfactory experiences during the hospital stay, so all it took was one more encounter to trigger their anger. Although this was the first time the afternoon nurse had met the family, his was the last in a series of interactions between the patient and the healthcare system that caused this family grief. Now, if the patient complains to the manager about this nurse, what can the manager do? If the manager does not have an appreciation for the nonlinear nature of systems, she may be tempted to discipline the nurse. However, if the manager does have an appreciation for the nonlinear nature of systems, she may try to re-create with the family the sequence of events. Although each event was relatively harmless considered individually, when linked together with the family's situation they contributed to a dissatisfying experience. From this investigation, the manager may identify areas that can be improved to enhance the patient's overall experience with the care-delivery process.

Another example of the nonlinear nature of systems may be seen in strategies used to reduce personnel expense in healthcare organizations. Because personnel expenses make up such a large percentage of operating budgets, changing the staff mix—that is, reducing the number of professional staff (e.g., registered nurses, medical technologists, pharmacists) and increasing the proportion of assistive personnel (e.g., nurses' aides, laboratory assistants, pharmacy technicians)—is a common cost-cutting intervention. When this intervention is studied from a systems perspective, however, the resulting sequences of activities and their interrelationships are more readily seen. The unplanned consequences of this cost-cutting strategy in one organization included an increase in the overall employee turnover rate because of the high turnover among the entry-level, assistive personnel group. Because this cost-cutting strategy was used by managers across different types of professions and departments, the stress and cost of continuously recruiting, hiring, and training new employees more than offset the savings hoped for from lowering the average hourly wage. When viewed from one department's point of view, the cost-reduction strategy may appear to be reasonable;

however, when the compounding effect of this cost-cutting strategy is viewed across the entire organization, the strategy designed to reduce costs actually undermines the organization's ability to do so (Kelly 1999).

Summary

Like the term "quality," the term "system" can carry a variety of connotations. In this text, a system refers to a collection of parts that interact with each other to form an interdependent whole, and systems thinking acknowledges the large number of parts in a system, the infinite number of ways in which the parts interact, and the nature of the interactions. The five system characteristics contributing to the presence of dynamic complexity are change, trade-offs, history dependency, tight coupling, and nonlinearity.

Exercise

Objective: To practice identifying dynamic complexity.

Instructions:
Describe how the following examples illustrate dynamic complexity.

Example 1:
"Hurricane Katrina devastated economies, communities, families and individuals along the US Gulf coast in 2005. Although the levees in New Orleans were known to be vulnerable (Fischetti 2001), policymakers chose *not* to invest the resources needed to strengthen them. The failure of the levees and the flooding that followed have led to the most expensive urban recovery and rebuilding effort in US history. Federal dollars that now must rebuild the shattered coast are no longer available to fund daycare centers, school lunch programs, Medicaid or nursing research. People fleeing from the Gulf coast evacuated to communities throughout the United States. On arrival in places such as Atlanta and Houston, they needed health services and replacement of essential prescription drugs—and most had no health records or insurance information . . . documents that would normally be essential."

From: Mason, K. D., J. K. Leavitt, and M. W. Chaffee. 2007. "Policy & Politics: A Framework for Action." In *Policy & Politics in Nursing and Health Care*, edited by K. D. Mason, J. K. Leavitt, and M. W. Chaffee, 1–20. St. Louis, MO: Elsevier.

Example 2:
"Hospitals nationwide are tangling with Wall Street to get out of disastrous wages that have complicated their financial problems. Some hospitals are paying millions of dollars in penalties to get out of derivatives contracts, after betting incorrectly that interest rates would rise. Other hospitals are paying

higher interest rates. At many, these ill-fated financial bets have contributed to layoffs and scuttled projects. More than 500 nonprofit hospitals—at least one in six—bought interest-rate "swaps" to lower their borrowing costs . . . the swaps allowed hospitals to act much like homeowners switching from a floating-rate mortgage to a fixed-rate one, betting on rising interest rates . . . these bets backfired when the Federal Reserve cut interest rates to nearly zero from more than 5% in 2007. . . . Financial engineering by Wall Street has been a huge part of hospitals' problems and has even translated into a lack of hospital beds."

From: Dugan, I. J. 2010. "Wrong-Way Financial Bets Have Hit Hard." *The Wall Street Journal*, July 10.

Companion Readings

Association of Academic Health Centers. 2008. "Out of Order Out of Time: The State of the Nation's Workforce." Washington, DC: Association of Academic Health Centers. [Online article; retrieved 1/17/11.] www.aahcdc.org/policy/AAHC_OutofTime_4WEB.pdf

Coutou, D. L. 2003. "Sense and Reliability: A Conversation with Celebrated Psychologist Karl E. Weick." *Harvard Business Review* 81 (4): 84–90.

Senge, P. M. 1990. "The Leader's New Work: Building Learning Organizations." *Sloan Management Review* (Fall): 149–65. (Note: This a classic article and has been reprinted in 1998 and 2006.)

Weick, K. E., and K. M. Sutcliffe. 2001. *Managing the Unexpected: Assuring High Performance in an Age of Complexity*, 1–23. San Francisco: Jossey-Bass.

Web Resources

Applied Systems Thinking: http://appliedsystemsthinking.com/
New England Complex Systems Institute (NECSI): www.necsi.edu/about/
Society of Organizational Learning: www.solonline.org/
System Dynamics Society: www.systemdynamics.org

UNDERSTANDING SYSTEM BEHAVIOR: SYSTEMIC STRUCTURE

Learning Objectives

After completing this chapter you should be able to:

- explain systemic structure from the perspective of the iceberg metaphor;
- explain the role of systemic structure in the sustainability of improvement interventions;
- describe how an understanding of systemic structure guides managerial questions about performance problems;
- explain how managers can develop their skills in recognizing systemic structure; and
- describe the influence of mental models on managerial behaviors, decisions, and effectiveness.

O n Thursday, Nurse Smith volunteers to work a double shift in the ICU. The next day, he misses his regularly scheduled shift when he calls in sick. The following month, Nurse Jones, who works in the same ICU, volunteers to work a double shift. Two days later, she misses her regularly scheduled shift when she calls in sick. When the ICU manager mentions this "coincidence" to two colleagues, they also describe similar situations on their respective units. As the ICU manager gathers more information about employee staffing practices, he realizes that although the policies help staffing in the short term, the same policies inadvertently contribute to increased sick calls and more overtime in the long run.

The manager discovers that well-intended efforts such as the carefully written policies and procedures for his department may not yield the expected results. Likewise, well-intended change or improvement interventions often yield disappointing results. This chapter explores how better understanding the dynamics of system behavior can help managers plan and execute improvement interventions in their organizations.

A Systems Metaphor for Organizations

Metaphors provide a concrete picture of a theoretical concept. Thinking of an organization as an iceberg is one metaphor that illustrates the subtle but

EXHIBIT 3.1
The Iceberg
Metaphor

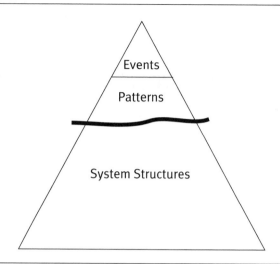

Source: Reprinted with permission from Innovation Associates, Inc. 1995. "Systems Thinking: A Language for Learning and Action." Participant manual, version 95.4.1. Waltham, Massachusetts.

powerful systems principles at work in organizations (Innovation Associates, Inc. 1995). Those forces that cause an organization to function the way it does and the people in the organization to behave the way they do are like the nine-tenths of an iceberg hidden underwater (NSIDC 2011). The essence of an organization is not visible to most observers; what is below the organizational "waterline" can undermine well-intended change initiatives, improvement efforts, and clinical interventions, just as the part of the iceberg beneath the water's surface can sink a passing ship.

The triangular shape in Exhibit 3.1 represents the iceberg, and the wavy, thick line represents the waterline. The tip of the iceberg (the top layer of the triangle) represents the events that occur daily in the organization. The middle layer of the iceberg represents a deeper understanding of the organization as a system that links events into patterns of behavior. The bottom level of the iceberg, which is underwater, represents the deepest understanding of the behavior of the organization as a system. This level represents relationships among system variables that cause the events and patterns to occur.

In the staffing example at the beginning of this chapter, the nurse managers saw the nurses working double shifts and calling in sick as unique events on each of their units. However, while comparing notes, they identified a pattern of similar behavior across their three different patient care units. Although the act of identifying patterns is above the organizational waterline, it is the first step toward systems thinking. The manager began to go below the waterline when he starting linking his observations into patterns. By telling a "story" of his discoveries, the relationships and underlying causes of the problems began to emerge. This was the story:

The hospital policies were supposed to promote adequate staffing and discourage sick calls; however, the day shifts were often over-staffed and the evening and nights shifts were understaffed.

Nurses were paid overtime and often an additional "premium" for working a double shift. When nurses volunteered for a double shift, they were positively perceived as "helpful" and "team players." The nurses helped out with a shift that was short-staffed and did not, in turn, cause staffing difficulties on their day shift by calling in sick.

By working a double shift and calling in sick later in the week, the nurses were able to work the same amount of hours but get paid more than if they had worked their regular scheduled shifts.

The manager began to identify the key system variables at work: scheduling policies, individual employee incentives and compensation, infor-mal rewards, sick-call policy, individual unit operations, and floatpool opera-tions. Although individually the policies and operations seemed reasonable, their interactions contributed to the underlying systemic structure. The per-ceived benefit to nurses (i.e., the opportunity to help out peers and patients and earn more money while working the same hours) and the frequency of nurses volunteering for a double shift and calling in sick later in the week were related in a way that reinforced the behavior—that is, as the number of nurses who perceived this benefit increased, the number of times the behavior occurred increased. Note that the nurses had no malicious intent in this case; they were simply following the policies as they were crafted. As this reinforcing relationship occurred across several nursing departments, an overall increase in salary expense became the unintended consequence to the hospital.

When the manager understood each of the policies within the con-text of how they made up the human resources system, he and the other managers were able to redesign the system to achieve the intended result of staffing the hospital in a dependable and cost-effective manner. Some of the changes this organization made to break the reinforcing cycle included reviewing the distribution of nurses during the day, evening, and night shifts to better balance staffing across the 24-hour period; improving coordina-tion between the nursing unit schedules and the floatpool's schedules; and changing the overtime criteria (consistent with legal labor requirements) from hours worked in excess of 8 hours per day to hours worked in excess of 40 hours per week.

Lessons for Healthcare Managers

In the iceberg metaphor for organizations, above-the-waterline activities are daily events and the patterns comprising these events. The term **systemic**

Systemic structure involves the inter-relationships among key ele-ments within the system and the influence of these interrelationships on the system's behavior over time (Senge 2006)

structure refers to what is found below the waterline. The systemic structure involves the interrelationships among key elements within the system and the influence of these interrelationships on the system's behavior over time (Senge 2006). Systemic structure refers to interrelationships among elements, components, and variables that make up the system, not to interpersonal relationships among people (Senge 2006). Systemic structure should also be differentiated from **organizational structure**, which refers to how responsibility and authority are distributed throughout an organization (Shortell and Kaluzny 2006), although organizational structure may act as a systemic structure.

Organizational structure
how responsibility and authority are distributed throughout an organization (Shortell and Kaluzny 2006)

Understanding systemic structure helps a manager to better understand the organization. Based on this understanding, the manager may choose high-leverage interventions to improve the organization's performance. Valuable insights about one's organization may be gained by understanding the concept of systemic structure. This section offers four lessons for healthcare managers:

1. Systemic structure influences behavior.
2. Systemic structure is not readily visible.
3. Information is essential to identifying systemic structure.
4. Successful change requires going below the waterline.

Lesson 1: Systemic Structure Influences Behavior

Consider the following story from an anonymous author:

> A college student spent an entire summer going to the football field every day wearing a black-and-white striped shirt, walking up and down the field for ten or fifteen minutes, throwing bird seed all over the field, blowing a whistle, and then walking off the field. At the end of the summer, it came time for the first home football game. The referee walked onto the field and blew the whistle. The game had to be delayed for a half hour to wait for the birds to get off the field.

Everyone laughs at this story. However, if one were sitting in the stadium stands without a clue about the events of the summer, one would probably be annoyed and blame those darn birds. The birds were not right or wrong. They were doing what they were supposed to be doing based on the underlying systemic structures: the relationships between feeding time and the football field, the striped shirt and the birdseed, the whistle and their hunger.

"Every organization is perfectly designed to get the results that it gets. To get different results you need to improve the design of the organization" (Hanna 1988, 36). This expression has almost become cliché in quality improvement presentations and articles. However, what is not commonly heard or read is that improvement designs must be targeted below the waterline, not simply above the waterline. An understanding of the iceberg metaphor prompts improvement questions to be asked from all levels of the iceberg to reveal the underlying structures that cause the patterns and events to occur.

Consider how the improvement interventions change depending on the level from which the improvement questions are asked. An events-level improvement question focuses on: "What does the individual need to do differently?" and usually results in the desire to blame an individual in response to unsatisfactory performance or a medical error. A patterns-level question moves from the individual to the group and focuses on: "What do we need to do differently?" Interventions at this level may target the collective actions of a team, a department, or an organization and may include implementing clinical guidelines, streamlining office scheduling systems, or installing new computers. The below-the-waterline question focuses on: "How can we best understand why we are getting the results we are getting?"(Exhibit 3.2).

The iceberg metaphor adds insight to issues on an industry level and on the organizational level. For example, in the 1990s, changing work conditions resulting from hospital restructuring and downsizing led nurses in Victoria, Australia, to change from

> full-time to part-time work because they couldn't cope with the strain of working full-time . . . because hospitals were having trouble getting nurses to work for them, temporary agencies stepped in to fill the gap. But this simply exacerbated the shortage. . . . Agencies were paying their nurses three times the amount of money permanent staff were getting . . . so more and more nurses left permanent work in the hospital and went and worked agency. . . . [I]nstead of rewarding permanent nurses to fill in schedule deficits,

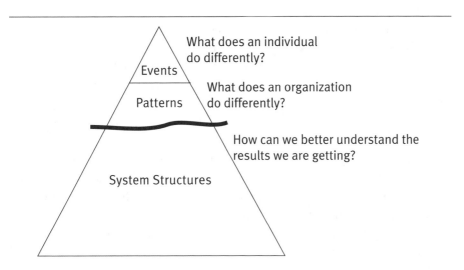

EXHIBIT 3.2

Improvement Questions

nurse managers were going to agency nurses. . . . [T]he permanent staff saw that the agency nurse was getting flexibility, shifts they wanted to work, and also more pay. So they left permanent work for agency work. . . . [C]osts of agency nurses rose from $30 million to $55 million a year. (Gordon 2005, 346)

Similar relationships among healthcare restructuring, work conditions, temporary agencies, and management philosophies have explained nationwide nurse shortages in the United States, Canada, and the United Kingdom (Gordon 2005).

Lesson 2: Systemic Structure Is Not Readily Visible

Systemic structure is not readily visible unless a conscious effort is made to find it. Just because managers do not see what is below the organizational waterline does not mean that systemic structure is not present in the organization. For example, a newly hired manager at an academic medical center was assigned to facilitate an improvement project on one patient care unit. If the project proved successful on this unit, the intent was to expand the intervention organization-wide. Despite positive results—as measured by improved cycle times, increased patient satisfaction, and increased staff satisfaction—the project was not implemented beyond the original pilot site. When the manager began to explore possible reasons that the project was not replicated on the other units, he discovered that over the years numerous project teams had designed and implemented successful pilot projects aimed at improving specific problems. However, few of these projects had actually been integrated into the ongoing activities of the organization (i.e., institutionalized).

Upon further investigation, he uncovered the following systemic structures operating in this organization. First, all improvements in the organization were called "pilots." The expectation was that a trial would be conducted for a specified period, that results would be presented to the administrative team, and that the administrative team would then authorize the project to continue or not. The problem was that this process occurred independently from the budgeting process. When the "special pools" of dollars to fund pilot initiatives were gone, no mechanisms were in place to reallocate funds either within or among departments to support a successful improvement or innovation.

The label of "pilot" also brought with it other short-term perceptions related to support, staffing, and budgets. Because of these hidden, but real, relationships among the variables required to support change, this academic medical center demonstrated a constant stream of successful improvement pilot efforts yet sustained improvement in the overall organizational performance never occurred.

Lesson 3: Information Is Essential to Identifying Systemic Structure

A *pattern* is defined as "a regular or repetitive form, order, or arrangement" (Encarta 2011). This definition implies that identifying or recognizing a pattern requires more than one observation. In the nurse staffing example, the discussion among the nurse managers about issues on their respective units provided an opportunity to observe behavior of many nurses across multiple units. Only when these observations were combined did the organizational pattern become evident.

The need for multiple observations or data points has implications for how managers determine reporting relationships, how they interact and communicate, and how they present performance data. The traditional vertical organizational structure, which compartmentalizes groups within rigid reporting lines, reduces the opportunity to interact across departments and disciplines and reduces the opportunity to identify organizational patterns.

Communication methods based on "telling" rather than "sharing" information also reduce the opportunity to identify organizational patterns by reducing two-way communication and the "fresh eyes" often needed to interpret and link events. Data reported by single time periods only (e.g., monthly departmental financial reports) reduce managers' ability to identify patterns over time in their own departments; on the other hand, aggregated organizational data reduce managers' opportunity to identify patterns across smaller units of analysis within the organization.

Strategies that can promote pattern identification and prompt investigation into underlying structures include:

- organizational structures and cultures that encourage interaction among levels and units,
- open and free flow of information, and
- performance data displayed graphically and plotted as run charts over time to make data trends over time more visible.

Lesson 4: Successful Change Requires Going Below the Waterline

To implement successful and lasting change efforts, managers must go below the organizational waterline. The iceberg metaphor explains why the potential of many change or improvement efforts is not fully realized. If changes are targeted at the event or pattern levels (i.e., what we do) rather than at the systemic structure level (i.e., what causes the system to behave the way it does), the effect will only be temporary. Because structure influences behavior, the only way to truly change behavior within the system is to identify, target, and change the underlying structures.

Many ideas have been proposed on how to improve organizational systems; however, a common challenge for managers and care providers alike is how to actually implement these ideas. Organizational culture may be thought of as an underlying systemic structure. The influence of hospital culture on the ability to convert CQI concepts into effective implementation has been described in the healthcare research literature (Shortell et al. 1995). Health services researchers have studied the role of systemic structures, such as leadership, context, and incentives, in guideline implementation (McCormack et al. 2002; Solberg 2000a, 2000b). These types of studies have helped to inform policy changes at the national level that target underlying structures and are discussed more in Chapter 8.

Going Below the Waterline

The captain of a ship sailing in the North Atlantic uses radar, sonar, and a bow watch (a sailor posted at the front of the ship to look out for danger) to alert him to underwater ice. Likewise, managers may also use strategies that alert them to underlying systemic structures. Following are three strategies managers may use:

1. Understanding history
2. Being aware of mental models
3. Integrating double-loop learning into their management philosophy and approach

Understanding History

History is a powerful underlying structure. A healthcare manager's current work may be influenced by her department's history, the hospital's history, a professional group's history, the community's history, or the industry's history. For example, the sudden death of a well-respected department manager had a long-lasting impact on the department staff. The new incumbent manager was faced not only with getting settled in a new role and new department but also with addressing the staff's grief. For new employees, the lack of shared history with the deceased manager was a source of polarization between the "before" and "after" staff and interfered with the entire staff's ability to achieve a high level of teamwork.

As another example, a physical therapist at a rehabilitation center that had recently been purchased by a for-profit organization carefully explained the organization's history to a patient's family. The previous owners and managers of the center were proud of their heritage of religious service and quality. The family inquired if their family member would still get what she needed at this for-profit facility, and the physical therapist informed the family that though the organization's ownership had changed, the staff still identified with the center's historic values.

In the book *The Social Transformation of American Medicine*, Paul Starr (1982) describes the evolution of the US medical profession and physicians' roles from the eighteenth century through the twentieth century. Although one may agree or disagree with Starr's conclusions, this book explains how the history of physicians, hospitals, and insurance companies shaped the healthcare industry of today, and as such the book provides an explanation of the current state of our healthcare system. Understanding the circumstances surrounding the Flexner report, which was published in 1910 and describes the state of medical education at the time, can provide insights into why medical schools are structured the way they are and into the role of academic medical centers in US healthcare (Starr 1982).

On a larger scale, the ability to achieve consensus around health reform in the United States is complicated by many factors. Understanding the historical evolution of the US healthcare system, the traditions of the American people upon which the US healthcare system is based, and the numerous occasions that national health insurance has been on the political agenda (1917, the 1930s, and the 1940s), can provide insights into systemic sources of controversy surrounding the Patient Protection and Affordable Care Act signed by President Obama on March 23, 2010 (Starr 1982; Kaiser Family Foundation 2005).

The simplest strategies that managers may use to understand history are to ask, listen, and read. In addition, large-group "visioning" meetings have incorporated structured discussions about history (Weisbord and Janoff 2010). Managers, especially those assuming a new role, may gain valuable insights by facilitating similar discussions with staff in their own departments. The following guidelines may help:

- Ask the group to identify significant events during defined periods. Events within the department, organization, community, clinical specialty or profession, or industry may be identified.
- List the events by periods of time (e.g., in five- or ten-year increments, depending on the group).
- Look for patterns in the listed events.

For example, one group of nurses in the postpartum area identified this event in their history discussion: At 5:00 every morning, the charge nurse would announce over the unit's intercom system, "Patients who have not had a bowel movement yet, please put on your nurse call light." The group burst into laughter, and one nurse observed, "Glad those 'good old days' are gone!" This simple observation helped the group let go of its resistance to a proposed change on the unit as it realized that it had experienced numerous changes over the years, most of which had direct benefit to the patients.

A manager in a laboratory was intrigued about the type of events identified during a history discussion with staff. Most of the identified events focused on current events from the news, and few events focused on

Cognitive psychology
the branch of psychology "concerned with all forms of cognition—the mental activities involved in acquiring and processing information—including attention, perception, learning, memory, thinking, problem-solving, decision-making and language" (*Dictionary of Psychology Online.* 2009a)

Schema
a "mental representation of some aspect of experience, based on prior experience and memory, structured in such a way as to facilitate (and sometimes to distort) perception, cognition, the drawing of inferences, or the interpretation of new information in terms of existing knowledge" (*Dictionary of Psychology Online* 2009b)

laboratory technology or the department, as he had anticipated. The manager realized that because the demographic composition of his department had been changing over the years (the technologists were 50 years old or older, the technical assistants and phlebotomists were 30 years old or younger), the two distinct demographics had little in common but current events. This realization helped to explain why previous team-building sessions had only been moderately successful and prompted the manager to establish common ground for his employees through a shared vision for the department. This manager also became more attentive to age diversity, succession planning, and the needs of differing demographic groups, particularly in his approaches to recruitment and hiring (Kelly 1999).

Being Aware of Mental Models

The field of **cognitive psychology** is the branch of psychology "concerned with all forms of cognition—the mental activities involved in acquiring and processing information—including attention, perception, learning, memory, thinking, problem-solving, decision-making and language" (*Dictionary of Psychology Online* 2009a). Within the field, the term **schema** refers to a "mental representation of some aspect of experience, based on prior experience and memory, structured in such a way as to facilitate (and sometimes to distort) perception, cognition, the drawing of inferences, or the interpretation of new information in terms of existing knowledge" (*Dictionary of Psychology Online* 2009b). In the management domain, the related term "**mental model**" is often used interchangeably with the terms "paradigm" and "assumption." Although these terms are technically slightly different, they all refer to a deeply ingrained way of thinking that influences how a person sees and understands the world and how that person acts. When someone declares an unquestionable status or condition, a mental model is usually being expressed; words like "always" and "never" are clues that mental models are being expressed. Mental models may be so strong that they override the facts at hand. For example, at a quality manager workshop, one hospital manager stated her mental model as follows: "Physicians would never spend time at a workshop like this." However, sitting beside her for the duration of the workshop were two pediatricians and a family practitioner!

What this manager did not realize was that her own mental model was interfering with her ability to design appropriate strategies to engage physicians in improvement efforts in her organization. As a result of her mental model, she found numerous reasons why physicians would not participate and was blinded to strategies to encourage physician participation. To promote learning and improvement in organizations, managers, care providers, and other employees in the organization must "look inward . . . to reflect critically on their own behavior, identify ways they often inadvertently contribute to the organization's problems, and then change how they act" (Argyris 1991). Without an understanding of our own mental models, we run the risk of unknowingly undermining our efforts to progress along the quality continuum.

Mental model
a deeply ingrained way of thinking that influences how a person sees and understands the world as well as how that person acts

For example, the mental model of "clinical guidelines are used to control physician behavior" encourages organizations to adopt top-down mandates for "cookbook" processes. Alternatively, the mental model "using evidence-based clinical guidelines to standardize steps of care can actually save physician time on routine interventions so that more time can be spent on the unique needs of the patient" encourages organizations to support and foster clinician involvement in evaluating, selecting, adapting, and implementing clinical guidelines. The mental model of "data are necessary to 'name, blame, and shame'" encourages managers to use data to justify punitive actions. The mental model of "information is power" encourages managers to guard data tightly and to distribute them only on a "need to know" basis. Alternatively, the mental model of "data are the foundation of performance improvement" encourages organizations to put in place information collection, analysis, and dissemination systems that make data easily accessible. Once mental models and their subsequent actions are understood, managers may purposely choose to operate from mental models that help rather than hinder in achieving desired performance results.

Differing mental models may also be a source of conflict within an organization. A manager's view or perspective on organizations themselves will shape her management strategies, actions, and style. Two contrasting views of organizations are the rational model and political model, which are shown in Exhibit 3.3 and are illustrated in the following example.

A manager who viewed organizations through a rational model was extremely frustrated with and ineffective in an organization that operated from a political perspective. From the manager's point of view, the decision-making processes in this politically driven organization served the interest of the players involved but did not result in optimal patient outcomes or cost-effective approaches. On the other hand, the administrative team perceived this manager's emphasis on results as interfering with the delicate political alliances they had worked hard to establish. The lack of understanding of each other's mental models created ongoing conflict between the manager and the administrative team: The manager thought the team did not care about results, and the team thought the manager was compromising relationships with important stakeholders. Without an awareness of each other's mental models, the conflict between the manager and the administrators continued to grow until the manager finally left the organization.

Had both parties made their mental models explicit—through discussion, definition of organizational operating principles, or orientation of new managers to the culture of decision making—their conflict may have been avoided, or at least some common understanding may have been established. Instead, the results were conflict, tension, and, eventually, manager turnover.

EXHIBIT 3.3
Comparison of
Organization
Models

Organizational Characteristic	Rational Model	Political Model
Goals, preferences	Consistent across members	Inconsistent, pluralistic within the organization
Power and control	Centralized	Diffuse, shifting coalitions and interest groups
Decision process	Logical, orderly, sequential	Disorderly, give and take of competing interests
Information	Extensive, systematic, accurate	Ambiguous, selectively available, used as a power resource
Cause-and-effect relationships	Predictable	Uncertain
Decisions	Based on outcome-maximizing choice	Result from bargaining and interplay among interests
Ideology	Efficiency and effectiveness	Struggle, conflict, winners and losers

Source: From Shortell, S. M. *Healthcare Management,* 4E. © 2000. Delmar Learning, a part of Cengage Learning, Inc. Reproduced by permission. www.cengage.com/permissions.

Double-loop learning
In double-loop learning, if one is not satisfied with the results or consequences, before taking action, underlying assumptions are examined, clarified, communicated, and/or reframed based on what the assumptions reveal. Only then is subsequent action, based on lessons revealed, taken (Argyris 1991; Tagg 2007)

Integrating Double-Loop Learning

A technique used to bring attention to mental models is double-loop learning. Exhibit 3.4 illustrates the difference between single- and double-loop learning. In single-loop learning, if one is not satisfied with the results or consequences of the actions, the actions are changed; however, the new actions are still driven by the same assumptions. In **double-loop learning**, if one is not satisfied with the results or consequences, underlying assumptions are examined, clarified, communicated, and/or reframed. Only then is subsequent action, based on lessons revealed, taken (Argyris 1991; Tagg 2007).

In one large hospital, a nursing supervisor complained to the manager of environmental services that when asked, the housekeeper refused to move a piece of equipment to prepare a room for a patient admission. The supervisor accused the housekeeper of being uncooperative and an obstacle to patient care. The supervisor operated from a professional mind-set and believed the housekeeper should be able to determine when the medical equipment may be touched. However, because of language, cultural, and educational differences among staff in entry-level positions, the environmental services staff were trained to strictly adhere to the department's standard policies and procedures, which stipulated that nurses' equipment not be disturbed. The housekeeper was operating from one set of assumptions (i.e., following the rules), while the nursing supervisor was operating from a conflicting set of assumptions (i.e., doing whatever needs to be done to care for the patient). Although both parties were trying to do their jobs the best way they knew, their opposing assumptions led to conflict and antagonism.

This situation of "accidental adversaries" may be unintentionally created when underlying assumptions are not known. The numerous roles, backgrounds, personalities, levels of education, and other diverse characteristics of the healthcare workforce necessitate managers to use double-loop learning to promote teamwork and quality within their scope of responsibility. In the workplace, however, managers often spend more time trying to mend adversarial relationships than prevent them. Managers may minimize accidental adversaries by:

- clarifying operating principles,
- helping staff understand and communicate their own assumptions,
- helping staff ask for clarification and explanations of others' behavior, and
- explicitly describing their (the managers') own expectations for individual employees and for teams.

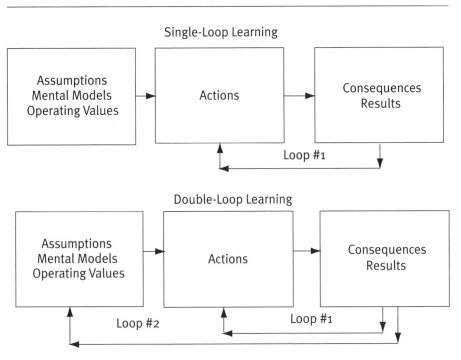

EXHIBIT 3.4

Single-Loop and Double-Loop Learning

Source: Adapted from Tagg, J. 2007. "Double-Loop Learning in Higher Education." *Change* 9 (4): 36–41. © 2007. Taylor & Francis Group. www.informaWorld.com

Double-loop learning is not appropriate for all situations in a health services organization. For example, an emergency resuscitation is not the time to question why a cardiac arrest code is carried out in a certain manner. While efficiency and consistency in day-to-day operations are accomplished through minimizing variation in how processes are carried out, double-loop learning should be an integral part of efforts that require innovative solutions or that require improved levels of performance. Managers and teams should be comfortable asking themselves and others questions such as, "Why do we do things the way we do? Is there a better way to get the job done? Are my own mental models helping or hurting my and our team's/department's/ organization's effectiveness?"

For an improvement team, double-loop learning may take the form of discussions that question "whether operating norms are appropriate—then inventing new norms as needed" (Pierce 2000, 15). Innovative solutions, such as the trigger tool approach to adverse drug events (Classen et al. 2008) and the Emergency Severity Index approach to emergency department triage (Gilboy et al. 2005), result from the process of double-loop learning. Managers may consider assigning a team member to be the "devil's advocate" and present an opposing view to ensure that assumptions are tested and challenged; otherwise, the challenger may be viewed as a barrier to the team process.

Summary

Organizations may be compared to an iceberg where events and patterns in the organization are above the waterline and system structures are below the waterline. *Systemic structure* refers to interrelationships among elements, components, and variables that make up the system and not to interpersonal relationships among people. Understanding systemic structure and how to identify it assists managers to solve problems by altering system behavior. Otherwise, managers risk treating symptoms of a problem and seeing the problem return over time.

Exercise

Objective: To explore double-loop learning by describing how operating values influence results.

Instructions:
- Read the article: McGinnis, J. M., and W. H. Foege. 2004. "The Immediate vs. the Important." *JAMA* 291 (10): 1263–64.
- In this article, two different operating values for the health services industry as a whole are suggested. These values are shown in the table. Based on your general knowledge, differentiate how these two operating values lead to industry actions and results.

Operating Values	Actions	Results
Treat the leading causes of death		
Treat the *actual* leading causes of death		

Companion Readings

Kaiser Family Foundation. n.d. "History of Health Reform in the U.S.: Interactive Timeline." [Online information; accessed 12/6/10.] http://healthreform.kff.org/flash/health-reform-new.html

Kaiser Family Foundation (producer). 2005. "Medicare and Medicaid at 40." [Online video; published 7/26/05.] www.kff.org/medicaid/40years.cfm

Starr, P. 1982. *The Social Transformation of American Medicine: The Rise of a Sovereign Profession and the Making of a Vast Industry*, 235–89. Reading, MA: The Perseus Books Group.

Swenson, S. J., G. S. Meyer, E. C. Nelson, G. C. Hunt, D. B. Pryor, J. I. Weissberg, G. S. Kaplan, J. Daley, G. R. Yates, M. R. Chassin, B. C. James, and D. M. Berwick. 2010. "Cottage Industry to Postindustrial Care—The Revolution in Health Care Delivery." *New England Journal of Medicine* 362 (5): e12(1)–e12(3).

Web Resources

Pegasus Communications: www.pegasuscom.com

Future Search: www.futuresearch.net

VISUALIZING SYSTEM RELATIONSHIPS: MODELS FOR HEALTH SERVICES MANAGERS

Learning Objectives

After completing this chapter, you should be able to:

- recognize the value of system models in explaining system relationships;
- contrast four different system models;
- relate system influences to organizational performance, including medical errors; and
- identify and distinguish between basic types of human errors.

Just as a road map provides a picture of how places are connected in a geographic area, models can provide a picture for managers of how elements may be connected within and between systems. These models are valuable managerial tools for revealing and providing insight about systemic structure. Similar to one's preference for an electronic map from a GPS (global positioning system) over a paper map, managers may prefer one model over another depending on their work settings, backgrounds, and individual preferences. Numerous models provide healthcare managers with a picture of the organizational system in which they work to help them recognize, understand, and anticipate how the parts of the systems are related and interact to form the whole.

The most basic system may be characterized by three elements: input(s), a conversion process, and output(s). These elements are demonstrated visually in the simple diagram:

Input(s) → Conversion process → Output(s)

In a health services organization, examples of inputs are patients, personnel, supplies, equipment, facilities, and capital. Examples of conversion processes are diagnostic processes, clinical treatments, operational activities, and business management functions. Examples of outputs are a patient's health status and an organization's business performance.

EXHIBIT 4.1
Quality
Management
System

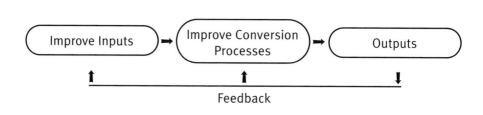

Feedback

Traditional quality efforts may be thought of in terms of managing the inputs and conversion process that comprise the system. Examples of ways to control the quality of personnel inputs include licensure requirements, continuing education, and performance appraisals. Examples of ways to control the quality of technology inputs such as drug therapies include clinical trials and US Food and Drug Administration (FDA) approval. Examples of ways to control the quality of a conversion process include clinical guidelines, process improvement, and standardization. Controlling the quality of the inputs and conversion processes is intended to improve the quality of the outputs, such as patient clinical and functional status, satisfaction with services, cost effectiveness, employee behaviors, and organizational culture.

Adding a feedback loop changes this basic system to a more dynamic one and, in turn, leads to a more mature approach to quality efforts. Feedback about the quality of the outputs guides efforts to improve the quality of the inputs and the conversion processes (Exhibit 4.1). Continuous feedback promotes continuous improvement. Viewing Donabedian's categories of medical quality measures and their relationship (structure → process → outcomes) mentioned in Chapter 1 in this light reveals the systems value of his perspective.

In Chapter 2, systems thinking is defined as "a discipline for seeing wholes. It is a framework for seeing interrelationships, rather than things, for seeing patterns of change rather that static 'snapshots'" (Senge 2006, 68). Improving the quality of the parts and understanding *and* improving the quality of the relationships between the parts lead managers to the most mature—or systems thinking—approach to quality management.

Four models to help managers view health services organizations within a systems context are presented in this chapter: the three core process model, the Baldrige Performance Excellence Program Health Care Criteria for Performance Excellence, the systems model of organizational accidents, and the socioecological framework.

Three Core Process Model

The three core process model shown in Exhibit 4.2 represents a "horizontal" view of a health services delivery organization; all processes in the organization

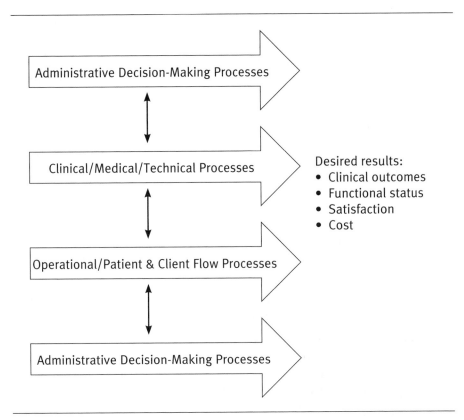

EXHIBIT 4.2
Three Core
Process Model

(represented by the arrows) should operate in an aligned fashion toward improving performance. The model starts on the right of the figure by defining desired results using a balanced set of outcomes: the patient's clinical outcomes, the patient's functional status, satisfaction, and cost of services.

In the three core process model the many processes that take place in a health services organization are grouped into three core categories: (1) clinical/medical/technical processes, (2) operational or patient flow processes, and (3) administrative processes.

Clinical/medical/technical processes are the fundamental reasons patients or clients seek the assistance of a health services organization—that is, to address some need that may be addressed by diagnosis, treatment, prevention, or palliative care. These processes include those under the domain of physicians and nonphysicians. The processes may be medical, such as surgery; mental-health related, such as counseling or therapy; related to daily care, such as nursing care after a stroke; or related to special treatments, such as obtaining oxygen or other durable medical equipment for the home.

Operational or patient flow processes enable a patient or client to access the clinical/medical/technical processes. This includes processes such as registering patients, scheduling activities, and coordinating services. Administrative decision-making processes occupy two positions in the figure, above and below the other two core processes. In this way, the model illustrates how administrative processes influence the overall organization. These processes include decision making, communication, resource allocation, and performance evaluation.

The arrows linking the three core processes reflect the interdependence of the processes.

Lessons for Healthcare Managers

The three core process model teaches managers several lessons. First, the interdependent relationships between the three core processes suggest that improvement in any one of these processes has the potential to increase the value of the service provided; however, the *concurrent* targeting of these core processes provides a synergy that can accelerate the achievement of improved outcomes. "An efficient clinical process supported by an inefficient operational process, or vice versa, is still an inefficient process. . . . [I]n addition, if . . . changes are made independent of clinician involvement, the likelihood of implementation is reduced. It is therefore necessary to have decision-making processes that actively engage clinicians in change efforts" (Kelly et al. 1997, 127–28).

For example, in one ambulatory surgery unit, the patient postoperative length of stay—the time the patient leaves the operating room to the time the patient is discharged—was found to be longer than in other, similar ambulatory surgery units. An improvement effort addressed the postoperative care process so that the discharge process could be improved and, in turn, the length of stay could be reduced. As the improvement effort progressed, the team realized that anesthesia practices were affecting their ability to achieve better results. If patients were being heavily sedated in the operating room and were slow to wake up as a result, the gains from improving the postoperative process could not be fully realized. Likewise, if the physicians implemented a new clinical protocol for anesthesia and pain management but patients still had to wait for the nurses to discharge them, gains from improving the anesthesia process could not be fully realized. Recognizing the interdependence of these two processes and targeting the discharge process *and* the anesthesia protocol for improvement allowed the benefits of both improvement efforts to be achieved. Furthermore, if the administrative processes did not permit employees to be scheduled away from clinical duties so they could be involved in the quality efforts, neither of the improvements could take place.

Second, the three core process model helps promote a patient-focused orientation by recognizing the need for aligning processes and improvement efforts toward the needs of the patient. The conceptual view of operations and administration observes how the patient (or client) moves through the entire system to access a clinical process. For example, a seemingly simple supervisory decision such as scheduling lunch breaks took on new meaning for one emergency department when the decision was viewed with patient flow in mind. Although scheduling staff lunch breaks at noon seemed reasonable, this practice created unnecessary patient delays and bottlenecks in the patient care processes because patient visits typically increased during the hours of 11:00 am to 1:00 pm. After ED management observed the situation from the patient flow perspective, the break policy was revised so that staff breaks occurred before and after—rather than during—busy patient times.

Third, the model reinforces the different yet necessary and interdependent contributions that each core process and each provider/implementer of those processes provide to patient care and organizational outcomes. This way, collaboration among the entire care team can be promoted.

Fourth, when the administrative role is viewed as a process rather than a function or a structure, the tools used to improve other types of processes may also be applied to administrative processes. If one of the desired outcomes is patient satisfaction, the administrative decision-making processes must include mechanisms to regularly collect, analyze, report, and evaluate patient satisfaction data and communicate these results throughout the organization.

The Baldrige Performance Excellence Program in Health Care Criteria

The Baldrige Performance Excellence Program's Health Care Criteria provide the most contemporary framework for organizational effectiveness, as described in Chapter 1 (Dean and Bowen 2000). For readers who desire a more in-depth explanation, a complete version of these criteria and examples of how health services organizations address the criteria may be found on the program's website (www.nist.gov/baldrige).

Exhibit 4.3 illustrates the essential elements in the model and the links between these elements. The following passage explains how to read and interpret the figure (National Institute of Standards and Technology 2011, 1):

> Your Organizational Profile (top of figure) sets the context for the way your organization operates. Your organization's environment, key working relationships, and strategic situation—including competitive environment, strategic challenges and advantages, and performance improvement system—serve as an overarching guide for your organizational performance management system.
>
> The performance system is composed of the six Baldrige Categories in the center of the figure that define your processes and the results you achieve.

EXHIBIT 4.3

Organizational
Profile for
Baldrige
Performance
Excellence
Program's
Framework for
Health Care

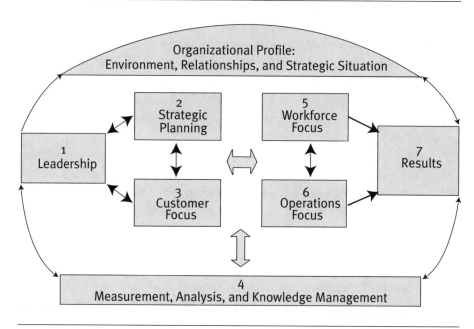

Source: National Institute of Standards and Technology (2011).

Leadership (Category 1), Strategic Planning (Category 2), and Customer Focus (Category 3) represent the leadership triad. These Categories are placed together to emphasize the importance of a leadership focus on strategy and on patients and stakeholders. Senior leaders set your organizational direction and seek future opportunities for your organization.

Workforce Focus (Category 5), Operations Focus (Category 6), and Results (Category 7) represent the results triad. Your organization's workforce and key operational processes accomplish the work of the organization that yields your overall performance results. All actions point toward Results—a composite of healthcare and process outcomes, customer-focused outcomes, workforce-focused outcomes, leadership and governance outcomes, and financial and market outcomes.

The horizontal arrow in the center of the framework links the leadership triad to the results triad, a linkage critical to organizational success. Furthermore, the arrow indicates the central relationship between Leadership (Category 1) and Results (Category 7). The two-headed arrows indicate the importance of feedback in an effective performance management system.

Measurement, Analysis, and Knowledge Management (Category 4) are critical to the effective management of your organization and to a fact-based, knowledge-driven system for improving healthcare and operational performance and competitiveness. Measurement, analysis, and knowledge management serve as a foundation for the performance management system.

Lessons for Healthcare Managers

Managers may take several lessons from the Baldrige systems model. First, the model describes the essential elements of organizational effectiveness (represented by the seven boxes in the model) and how they are related. The model recognizes the unique circumstances in which different organizations operate and encourages managers to base decisions, strategies, and interventions on their unique organizational profile. The overarching nature of the organizational profile promotes ongoing consideration of external influences, such as environmental, regulatory, or market demands.

When viewed in light of the Baldrige model, one can see that the principles of total quality (customer focus, continuous improvement, and teamwork), described in Chapter 1, touch on some required elements (customer focus, operations focus, and workforce focus) but not all of the required elements. The Baldrige model visually illustrates that a systems approach to quality management in a healthcare organization requires managers to focus attention not only on the three principles of total quality but also on the way the external operating environment, leadership, strategic planning, measurement, analysis and knowledge management, and a broader focus on the workforce contribute individually and collectively to achieving the desired organizational performance results.

For example, managers who use this model understand the importance of alignment within the organization. This means that the activities within each box in the model are directed toward achieving the same results and that organizational and management choices are consistent with the organization's mission, vision, values, strategic direction, and patient and stakeholder requirements. For example, one health services organization offers comprehensive quality improvement training for its managers. Each manager is expected to design and carry out an improvement effort as a requirement of the training, so each selects a topic on which to focus his improvement project. Although each manager demonstrates improvement in the chosen area, the collective improvements of all of the training participants may not contribute to the overall organizational objectives. This observation is illustrated by one manager who devoted much time and effort to improving a service area that was eliminated by the organization the following year. Another healthcare organization offering a similar type of training for managers used senior leaders to help the managers select improvement topics that would not only provide benefit within the managers' scope of responsibility but also would contribute to the overall organizational strategy.

The Baldrige model also illustrates the link between management and human resource needs. Before implementing a process improvement, managers ask themselves, "What needs to happen to ensure that the staff will succeed at implementing the new process?" As a result, when a new process is initially implemented, managers may need to give employees some leeway as they learn the new process or their new roles. Adapting to something new takes time, and by planning ahead, the manager may be able to negotiate for the short-term budget or productivity variance required for the transition period. An understanding of the Baldrige model helps managers realize that their role in process improvement also includes ensuring that employees have the information, training, and tools they need to successfully implement improvements in the work setting.

This model emphasizes the importance of alignment of data, analysis, and performance indicators. Managers using the Baldrige model choose performance indicators in a systematic way. When designing their performance measurement system and selecting performance indicators, managers consistently ask themselves the following series of questions (National Institute of Standards and Technology 2011):

- What are the key determinants of success for our setting of care?
- Who are our patients and stakeholders, and what are their requirements?
- How do these determinants and requirements guide decisions about our organizational goals?
- Are these goals consistent with the mission, vision, and values of the organization?
- What approach(es) will we use to meet our goals?
- What is the desired impact for selecting this particular approach?
- What performance indicators will allow us to measure the desired impact?
- How often should each of these indicators be reviewed, and by whom?
- What data collection, analysis, and reporting capabilities are necessary to deliver the performance indicators as determined?

Finally, the Baldrige model illustrates essential linkages within the system. The interrelationships between the system elements are represented by the arrows. Close attention to the location of the arrows and the direction of the arrowheads guides managers on key system feedback and communication loops. The arrows also help managers trace relationships throughout the system to gain insight about their contribution to organizational results.

Errors
"all those occasions in which a planned sequence of mental or physical activities fails to achieve its intended outcome" (Reason 1990, 9)

Adverse event
"an injury caused by medical management rather than the underlying condition of the patient" (IOM 1999, 4)

Violations
"deviations from safe operating practices, procedures, standards or rules" (Reason 1997, 72)

For example, one manager realized that in her organization, the large arrow connecting the leadership triad with the results triad was one-way only; communication flowed in one direction only with little opportunity for the managers and other staff to provide feedback for consideration in decision making at the organizational level. This realization helped to explain her perceived disconnect between organization-wide initiatives and her department's local circumstances and needs.

Systems Model of Organizational Accidents

James Reason's systems model of organizational accidents is intended to explain how medical errors may occur in health services organizations. This model not only takes into account the relationships between elements in the system, but it also integrates the characteristics of dynamic complexity described in Chapter 2.

To understand Reason's model, one must first understand the definitions and assumptions upon which it is based. **Errors** are defined as "all those occasions in which a planned sequence of mental or physical activities fails to achieve its intended outcome" (Reason 1990, 9). An **adverse event** is defined as "an injury caused by medical management rather than the underlying condition of the patient" (IOM 1999, 4). **Violations** are "deviations from safe operating practices, procedures, standards or rules" (Reason 1997, 72).

Errors may be further categorized as **judgment errors** (improper selection of an objective or a plan of action), **execution errors** (proper plan carried out improperly), **errors of omission** (something that should be done is not done), and **errors of commission** (something that should not be done is done) (Reason 1990; IOM 1999). **Active errors** are those committed by frontline workers; the results of active errors are usually seen immediately (Reason 1990, 1997). For example, a restaurant-server trainee picks up a hot plate by mistake, quickly lets it go, and watches the plate and its contents crash to the kitchen floor. **Latent errors**, on the other hand, occur in the upper levels of the organization. The error may lie dormant for days or years until a particular combination of circumstances allows the latent error to become an adverse event (Reason 1990, 1997).

Violations may also be further categorized as routine, optimizing, and situation. **Routine violations** may be thought of as cutting-corners activities. **Optimizing violations** are "actions taken to further personal rather than task related goals" (Reason 1995, 82). **Situation violations** occur when a person believes that the action "offer[s] the only path available to getting the job done and where the rules or procedures are seen as inappropriate for the present situation" (Reason 1995, 82).

Judgment errors
improper selection of an objective or a plan of action

Execution errors
proper plan carried out improperly

Errors of omission
something that should be done is not done

Errors of commission
something that should not be done is done

Active errors
errors committed by frontline workers; the results are seen immediately (Reason 1990, 1997)

Latent errors
errors occurring in the upper levels of the organization; the error may lie dormant for days or years until a particular combination of circumstances allows the latent error to become an adverse event (Reason 1990, 1997)

EXHIBIT 4.4
Errors versus
Violations

	Errors	Violations
Where	Cognitive domain (the mind)	Social domain (organizational context)
Why	Informational problem	Motivational problem
Prevention	Improve knowledge and information	Address motivational and organizational factors

Sources: Reason (1995); Kelly (2009a).

Routine violations
when a step in a
process is inten-
tionally skipped;
cutting-corners
activities

*Optimizing
violations*
"actions taken to
further personal
rather than task
related goals"
(Reason 1995, 82)

*Situation
violations*
occur when a
person believes
that the action
"offer[s] the only
path available to
getting the job
done and where
the rules or pro-
cedures are seen
as inappropriate
for the present
situation" (Reason
1995, 82)

The distinction between errors and violations is important to managers because they have different contributing causes and, in turn, require different solutions as summarized in Exhibit 4.4.

Finally, Reason's model assumes a collection of defenses that act as buffers or safeguards to prevent a hazardous situation from becoming an adverse event, just as a thick oven mitt would prevent the restaurant worker from dropping a hot dish. The collection of defenses in an organization may be thought of as several slices of Swiss cheese lined up next to each other. The holes in the slices of cheese represent the latent and active errors present in the organization. Even though an error may be present (i.e., a hole in one slice), it does not result in an adverse event or accident because there are organizational defenses to stop it from continuing (i.e., the next slice). The Joint Commission Standard MM.05.01.01 is based on this premise. This standard states that "a pharmacist reviews the appropriateness of all medication orders for medications to be dispensed in the hospital" (Joint Commission 2010). A physician may inadvertently write an incorrect dosage; however, when the pharmacist picks up the mistake and clarifies the order with the physician (organizational defense), a medical error and potential adverse event is prevented.

Exhibit 4.5 illustrates the slices of Swiss cheese (or collection of defenses). The exhibit shows that under certain circumstances, the interplay between latent errors, local conditions, and active errors causes the holes in the cheese to align just right so that a sequence of events may pass through all the holes and result in an adverse event.

Lessons for Healthcare Managers

Administrative and management professionals play key roles in medical errors, as they are the source of latent errors in organizations (Reason 1997, 10).

> Latent conditions are to technical organizations what resident pathogens are to the human body. Like pathogens, latent conditions—such as poor design, gaps in supervision, undetected manufacturing or maintenance failures, unworkable procedures, clumsy

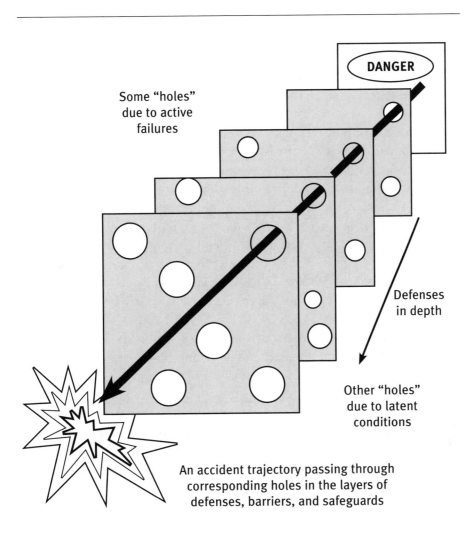

Some "holes" due to active failures

DANGER

Defenses in depth

Other "holes" due to latent conditions

An accident trajectory passing through corresponding holes in the layers of defenses, barriers, and safeguards

EXHIBIT 4.5

Systems Model of Organizational Accidents: Swiss Cheese Defenses

Source: © *Managing the Risks of Organizational Accidents.* Reason, J. 1997. Ashgate Publishing Limited. Reprinted with Permission.

automation, shortfalls in training, less than adequate tools and equipment—may be present for years before they combine with local circumstances and active failures to penetrate the system's many layers of defenses. They arise from strategic and other top-level decisions made by governments, regulators, manufacturers, designers and organizational managers. The impact of these decisions spreads throughout the organization, shaping a distinctive corporate culture and creating error-producing factors within the individual workplaces. . . . Latent conditions are an inevitable part of organizational life. Nor are they necessarily the products of bad decisions, although they may well be. Resources, for example, are rarely distributed equally between an organization's various departments. The original decision on how to allocate them may have been based on sound . . . arguments, but all such inequities create quality, reliability, or safety problems for someone, somewhere in the system at some later point.

Frontline employees or those in direct contact with patients, clients, and customers serve as the last layer of defense to prevent an error and the last layer where a defense may break down. While the results of a sequence of events leading to the medical error or adverse event occur at the point of patient contact, the causes may be found throughout all levels of the organization. Reason describes that the frontline staff, "rather than being the main instigators of an accident . . . tend to be the inheritors of system defects created by poor design, incorrect installation, faulty maintenance, and bad management decisions. Their part is usually that of adding the final garnish to a lethal brew whose ingredients have already been long in the cooking" (Reason 1990, 173).

Latent errors may occur at the level of senior leaders who design organizational goals and priorities and determine how human, financial, and capital resources are allocated. Latent errors may occur at the level of frontline managers who translate and implement senior-level goals and priorities within their own scope of responsibilities. Frontline management includes those responsible for departments that provide direct patient or client services; departments that maintain and support the environment in which services are provided and the tools used by providers; and departments that support the business functions of the organization. Decisions at the senior and frontline management levels of the organization, in turn, support preconditions for safe care in the form of appropriate, functioning, and reliable equipment; a knowledgeable, skilled, and trained workforce; appropriately designed work processes, communication mechanisms, and staffing plans; and effective supervision. Alternatively, decisions at these two levels of the organization may promote the preconditions of error-prone work environments and processes.

While Reason's model represents a general organizational model, Hofmann examines specific sources, causes, types, and examples of latent management errors in health services organizations. For example, "inadequate preparation of/by decision maker(s), political pressure, flawed decision-maker process, and ignorance of legitimate alternatives" are causes of errors within the managerial domain of health services organizations (Hofmann 2005, 10). Errors of omission include "failure to delegate and hold subordinates accountable; failure to consider all options; failure to balance power interests; and, failure to anticipate significant factors affecting decisions" (Hofmann 2005, 11). Errors of commission include "permitting decisions to be made without adequate analysis; choosing political, not business solutions;

withholding negative information from individuals with the right to know; and making economic decisions that harm clinical care and outcomes" (Hofmann 2005, 11). An understanding of Reason's model emphasizes the imperative for managers' evidence-based knowledge, skill, and abilities. By complementing safer practices of their clinical and technical counterparts, managers help safeguard the multiple levels of the organization in which errors may occur.

Socioecological Framework

The socioecological framework represents a transdisciplinary systems perspective on promoting health and wellness that uses and reflects theory from multiple fields including medicine, public health, and the behavior and social sciences. Stokols further describes the underpinnings of the socioecological framework.

> The healthfulness of a situation and the well-being of its participants are assumed to be influenced by multiple facets of both the physical environment (e.g., geography, architecture, and technology) and the social environment (e.g., culture, economics and politics). Moreover, the health status of individuals and groups is influenced not only by environmental factors but also by a variety of personal attributes, including genetic heritage, pyschological dispositions, and behavioral patterns. Thus, efforts to promote human well-being should be based on an understanding of the interplay among the diverse environmental, biological, or behavioral factors." (Stokols 2000, 27)

Key to this framework is the recognition of "the complexity of human environments" and the emphasis on multilevel, interrelated influences and multilevel, interrelated interventions influencing health and wellness (Stokols 2000). These multiple levels may be thought of as nested systems within systems starting with the individual and expanding to include "interpersonal, organization, community, society, supranational" (Kok et al. 2008, 438). Reed illustrates the multiple and interrelated levels of influences (determinants) and interventions in Exhibit 4.6. Reading the exhibit top to bottom illustrates the four levels of determinants of health behavior: individual, organization, community, and population (Reed 2001). Reading the exhibit left to right illustrates that for each of these levels of determinants, specific interventions may be implemented and their effect evaluated. For example, the model may be used to better understand smoking behavior.

Individual determinants of smoking behavior include a person's knowledge of associated health risks and the smoking behavior of family and friends. Individual interventions to reduce smoking behaviors may include smoking-cessation classes and pharmacotherapy (e.g., nicotine patches). The

EXHIBIT 4.6
Socio-
ecological
Framework

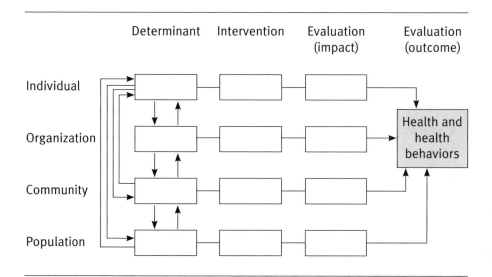

Source: This illustration reprinted with permission by Peter Reed, M.P.H., JoAnne Earp, Sc.D., and the instructors of HBHE 131, *Introduction to Social Behavior in Public Health,* Department of Health Behavior and Health Education, University of North Carolina at Chapel Hill, School of Public Health, 2001.

impact is measured by whether the person stops smoking or does not start in the first place.

Organization determinants of smoking behavior include policies regarding smoking in the workplace and the availability of smoking-cessation classes as an employee health benefit. Prohibiting smoking, offering limited access to on-site smoking areas, and reimbursing employees for smoking-cessation classes are interventions targeted at the organizational level. The proportion of employees who smoke and the "quit rate" are common organizational evaluation measures.

Community determinants of smoking behavior include social norms and beliefs. For example, smoking may be linked to social status and acceptance. Because of the history of tobacco farming in the southeastern United States, smoking has also been associated with the community's economic livelihood. Redefining social norms and recruiting nontobacco economic opportunities would be considered community-level interventions. Impact may be measured in terms of community smoking rates.

Population determinants of smoking behavior include regulations regarding smoking in public places. Interventions such as no-smoking airline flights, no-smoking buildings, or a "sin tax" on cigarettes are examples of population-level interventions. The effect may be measured by compliance with regulations and population smoking rates.

In Exhibit 4.6, the arrows between the levels indicate the interconnectedness of the determinants, interventions, and impact at all levels. While a level-specific intervention may be effective, recognizing the relationships between the levels creates a synergy to enhance desired outcomes. Using the example on smoking, one can understand the limited impact of enrolling a person in a smoking-cessation class when he is surrounded by smokers in the family, in the workplace, and in public venues.

Lessons for Healthcare Managers

The major lesson from this model for healthcare managers is that it provides a more expansive view of the nature of health and wellness in general and of health services specifically. In doing so, the model offers a larger context from which to understand interventions designed to improve the quality and safety of services provided by health services organizations and, in turn, understand complementary and competing interventions within and between levels.

In 2001, the Institute of Medicine recommended that "the changes needed to realize a substantial improvement in health care involve the health

Three Core Process Model	Baldrige Performance Excellence Program	Systems Models of Organizational Accidents	Socioecological Framework
Encourages concurrent improvement of interdependent processes	Shows how the components of performance excellence are related	Explains administrators and managers as sources of latent errors	Broadens and expands the manager's view
Aligns processes around patient/client/customer needs	Recognizes the context in which the organization operates	Describes frontline consequences of system errors	Addresses community and policy influences on health outcomes
Values all provider/employee groups	Promotes alignment of all activities within the organization	Emphasizes importance of management competence	Illustrates the interrelationships between multiple levels involved in leading to and improving health outcomes
Views administrative role as a process rather than a function	Promotes alignment of performance indicators	Distinguishes types of errors to appropriately design interventions	Encourages inter-related, multilevel interventions
	Illustrates essential links within the system		

EXHIBIT 4.7
Systems Models: Lessons for Managers

care system as a whole" (Institute of Medicine 2001a, 20). This recommendation implies understanding not only how organizations work as systems but also how the multiple players and layers involved in the health services industry are interrelated. The socioecological framework can help managers understand the increasing activity on the part of professional societies; regulatory agencies; and local, state, and federal governments to improve the quality and safety of healthcare.

Summary

As described in Chapter 3, systemic structures may not be readily visible. System models are valuable managerial tools to help managers identify elements and connections between those elements within their organizations and the environments in which they operate. Exhibit 4.7 summarizes lessons from the four system models discussed in this chapter. Managers are encouraged to identify, integrate, and continuously apply lessons from each of these models to further develop their skills in understanding systemic structures.

Exercise

Objective: To practice identifying different types of errors.

Instructions:
- Consider the following scenario:

   In Florida, Clara, an active 94-year-old great-grandmother who still worked as a hospital volunteer two days a week, was admitted to the hospital for a bowel obstruction. She and her family, along with nurses from the hospital, said that there were too few nurses to check her during the night when her eldest son went home to sleep for a couple of hours. Clara called the nurses to help her use the bathroom but when no one came, she climbed over the bed railing. Still groggy from surgery 20 hours earlier, Clara fell to the floor and broke her left hip. She died two days later during surgery to repair the hip fracture. "It was just too much for her," said her grandson. "For want of one nurse, she died" (Gibson and Singh 2003, 101).

- Review the following list of possible errors that could have been involved in this scenario.
   o One nurse and one nurse aide absent due to illness that night.
   o Clara's age.
   o No staff available to fill in for the two people calling in sick.
   o Falls risk assessment not completed on patient's chart.
   o Decision to upgrade CT scanner over modernizing patient beds.
   o Lack of training for nurses about specialized needs of elderly patients, especially related to their responses to medications.

○ Clara's son went home to sleep.

○ Night shift was consistently scheduled with the minimum staff needed on this unit.

○ Bioengineering had skipped last month's preventive maintenance check on the call light system because they were six weeks behind on their work.

○ Three new patients were admitted to this unit from the emergency department between 7:00 pm and 10:00 pm.

○ Falls precautions not implemented for this patient.

The above list includes latent errors, active errors, and preconditions. Write the errors in column 2 beside the appropriate category/type of failure.

Category/Type of Failure	Error
Latent error at the level of senior decision makers	
Latent failures at the level of frontline management	
Circumstances or conditions present when the patient's accident occurred	
Active errors associated with this event	

Companion Readings

Baldrige Performance Excellence Program. 2011. "2011–2012 Health Care Criteria for Performance Excellence." [Online information; retrieved 1/20/11.] www.nist.gov/baldrige/publications/hc_criteria.cfm

De Vries, E. N., M. A. Ramrattan, S. M. Smorenburg, D. J. Gouma, and M. A. Boermeester. 2008. "The Incidence and Nature of In-Hospital Adverse

Events: A Systematic Review." *Quality and Safety in Health Care* 17: 216–23.

Reiman T., E. Elina Pietikäinen, and P. Oedewald. 2010. "Multilayered Approach to Patient Safety Culture." *Quality and Safety in Health Care* 19: 1–5.

Van Beuzekom M., F. Boer, S. Akerboom, and P. Hudson. 2010. "Patient Safety: Latent Risk Factors." *British Journal of Anaesthesia* 105 (1): 52–59.

Web Resources

Federal Quality Program

Baldrige Performance Excellence Program: www.nist.gov/baldrige/

Baldrige Health Care Criteria for Performance Excellence: www.nist.gov/baldrige/publications/hc_criteria.cfm

Baldrige National Quality Award Winners (Healthcare)

Organizational profiles, contact information, and award application summaries: www.baldrige.nist.gov/Contacts_Profiles.htm

2010 Advocate Good Samaritan Hospital

2009 Heartland Health and VA Cooperative Studies Program Clinical Research Pharmacy Coordinating Center

2008 Poudre Valley Health System

2007 Mercy Health System

2006 North Mississippi Medical Center

2005 Bronson Methodist Hospital

2004 Robert Wood Johnson University Hospital, Hamilton

2003 Saint Luke's Hospital of Kansas City and Baptist Hospital, Inc.

2002 SSM Health Care

Additional Resources

Agency for Healthcare Research and Quality Patient Safety Network: www.psnet.ahrq.gov/

American Nurses Association National Center for Nursing Quality: www.nursingworld.org/quality/

Anesthesia Patient Safety Foundation: www.apsf.org/

National Patient Safety Foundation: www.npsf.org/

Veterans Administration National Center for Patient Safety: www.patientsafety.gov/

ACHIEVING QUALITY RESULTS IN COMPLEX SYSTEMS

ESTABLISHING SYSTEM DIRECTION

Learning Objectives

After completing this chapter you should be able to:

- link the role of mission, vision, and context to organizational results;
- describe the value of defining purpose;
- appreciate how the purpose principle can aid managers in problem solving;
- distinguish the relationships between purpose, desired results, measures of results, interventions, and improvement goals; and
- compare the concepts of mental model and context as they are used in organizations.

The quality department at Hospital A defines its mission as "Help departments improve their quality indicators and to meet regulatory requirements." The hospital has consistently met The Joint Commission standards requirements and has demonstrated improvement on the quality indicators required by The Joint Commission and by the Centers for Medicare & Medicaid Services (CMS); however, physicians at Hospital A consistently complain to the CEO about bottlenecks in scheduling x-ray examinations for their patients and delays in receiving results for just about any diagnostic test.

The quality department at Hospital B defines its mission as "Providing technical and consultative support to departments, managers, and teams to help them improve value to their customers." Hospital B also consistently meets The Joint Commission standards requirements and demonstrates improvement in The Joint Commission and CMS quality indicators. However, Hospital B also demonstrates improved cycle times in numerous clinical diagnostic processes and has reduced its overall operational costs and improved employee satisfaction and retention.

Organizations operating from the mature end of the quality continuum know that their mission is much more than a catchy slogan or a poster on the wall. The **mission** defines the system's identity. The mission statement is used to explain and communicate why the organization or department exists, what the department is organized to do, or what a group is trying to

Mission
statement that
defines the system's identity

Purpose
an identity or
reason for being

achieve. A clear and shared understanding of the system's identity is essential for sustainability and to successfully adapt to changing external demands in its operating environment. In this book, the identity or reason for being is referred to as **purpose**.

The quality department in Hospital A defined itself in terms of a narrow purpose ("help," "meet") and a singular goal ("improve"); the department was looking to attain specific results in accordance with defined performance indicators. Hospital A succeeded in achieving these results, but it was not successful in achieving an overall quality organization. In Hospital B, the quality department defined itself in a broader way that permitted flexibility in how it defined its goals, focus, and interventions. For example, departmental goals could include: "improve care delivered to those patient populations addressed by the indicators." A focus on improving the hospital's overall admission and discharge processes could improve not only the ability to identify patients at risk for pneumonia and administer pneumococcal and influenza immunizations before discharge (required indicators) but also the overall quality of the patient and family's transition from the acute care setting to home, home care, or long-term care (CMS 2010a, 2010b).

Managers should consciously and consistently question purpose at all levels of the organization—that is, the purpose of individual activities, roles, processes, departments, programs, and the organization overall. At the system level, purpose defines the system. A clear understanding of purpose guides managers in establishing direction for improvements, helps them know they are working on the right problems, and increases the likelihood that quality efforts will achieve intended results. Without a clear understanding of purpose, managers run the risk of wasting time and resources by working on the wrong problem or improving something that should not exist in the first place.

This chapter explores the concept of purpose and its importance for managers. Companion concepts of vision and context are also discussed.

Purpose

In Chapter 1, Donabedian's causal relationship of quality-of-care measures was described as "Structure → Process → Outcome." However, when designing or redesigning interventions to improve results, the sequence is conceptually reversed: a clear understanding of purpose should guide the way organizations define desired outcomes. The purpose and desired outcomes should guide the way processes are designed to support achieving that purpose, and the structure (how people are organized, roles are defined, and tools and technology are selected) should be guided by the requirements of the process. This sequence may be thought of as:

Purpose/Desired Outcomes → Process → Structure.

When using this conceptual sequence, understanding and clarifying purpose serve important roles in setting direction by defining why an entity exists. Discussions of purpose also ensure that the right problem is being addressed, common ground is fostered, and breakthrough ideas and solutions are promoted.

Setting Direction

A student's purpose or identity shapes his selection of classes. A student with an identity of musician may take music theory and instrument classes, whereas a medical student may choose anatomy and physiology classes. Similarly, the identity of an organization or a department shapes its management's choices of goals, priorities, resource allocation, and improvement targets.

A hospital-based laboratory performed tests for the inpatient and outpatient populations of the tertiary care hospital in which it was located and for smaller hospitals and physicians' offices in the area. The manager and medical director, faced with the need to redesign the laboratory's operations, set a departmental goal to redesign the processes and the work area to improve efficiency and better meet customer needs. To accomplish this they created a redesign team.

One of the first topics the redesign team discussed was the laboratory's purpose. Initially, the team described the laboratory's purpose as providing customer service. For a hospital that had formally adopted a total quality philosophy several years before, the team's focus on customer service indicated that they had integrated this total quality principle into their way of operating. However, to provide customer service was not a reason to exist; customer service was a part of what the laboratory provided but not its sole function. It was necessary to provide something other than customer service.

The improvement facilitator and the manager invited panels of internal customers to talk with the team about their expectations and experiences as customers of this laboratory's service. The common theme heard from each customer, whether a nurse in the emergency department or a doctor's office, was that they depended on the information the laboratory gave them to make patient care decisions. In their efforts to provide quality service, the laboratory had lost sight of the reason it existed: to provide information. The team realized that quality service was a desired characteristic in how they delivered the information.

As the team continued to discuss the laboratory's purpose, it also realized that they provided customers with three distinct types of information. The first type of information was clinical patient data in the form of test results. Within this "product line" were numerous types of results from many types of specimens, from blood for analyzing cholesterol levels to tissue for analyzing a cancerous tumor. Over the years, however, the laboratory's role had evolved in response to changing reimbursement schemes, new technology, and published research on clinical treatments and interventions. As a result, the laboratory provided its customers with two additional "product lines": (1) evidence to providers about how to use and interpret newly available tests and testing methods, and (2) information related to the technical and regulatory requirements that became important as tests moved away from the laboratory to point-of-care techniques carried out by nurses or physicians.

Clarifying its purpose became an empowering realization for the laboratory staff. Each of the three product lines of information was necessary to provide laboratory services to all of its customers; however, only one—clinical laboratory results—was a potential source of measurable revenue or expense for this department; the other two product lines were solely a source of expense for the department. Equipped with a clear definition of purpose and arguing with a systems point of view, the laboratory manager and medical director were able to negotiate budgetary expectations with their administrator. They were able to articulate that the laboratory may be incurring expenses that ultimately benefited the quality of patient care in other departments and reduced the cost of the patient's total hospital experience. The budget discussions changed from focusing exclusively on reducing laboratory expenses to including how to measure and preserve the laboratory's essential role in providing overall quality of laboratory services to all patients within its service domain, not simply for work carried out within the boundaries of the laboratory's walls (Kelly 1998).

Addressing the Right Problem

The manager in an ambulatory surgery unit was faced with the problem of frequent patient delays, which led to patient complaints and higher costs. The manager assembled a team to address the goal of improving patient flow to improve clinical outcomes, patient satisfaction, and cost effectiveness (Kelly et al. 1997).

In one of the first improvement team meetings, the improvement facilitator asked the team to identify the major phases of care that make up the entire process of care for a patient experiencing ambulatory surgery. The team identified five phases that an ambulatory surgery patient goes through: (1) the pre-admission phase—care occurring somewhere other than in the ambulatory surgery unit; (2) the preoperative phase—care occurring in the ambulatory surgery unit before the patient goes to the operating room; (3) the intraoperative phase—the actual operation taking place in the operating room; (4) the postoperative phase—care supporting patient recovery and taking place in the recovery room or the ambulatory surgery unit; and (5) the post-admission phase—care occurring after the patient is discharged from the ambulatory surgery unit; this may include a follow-up phone call by a nurse or follow-up care in the physician's office.

The facilitator then asked the team to select an area that, if improved, could have the biggest impact on improving patient flow and reducing delays. The team chose the pre-hospital phase because this process was "upstream" to all of the others. If delays or breakdowns occurred during this phase of care, the rest of the process would also be delayed.

Next, the facilitator led a discussion about the purpose of the pre-admission phase of care. Immediately the team replied, "To prepare the patient for surgery; to make sure the patient is ready." As the purpose discussion continued, the team had a breakthrough when they realized that, although the pre-admission phase of care helped to prepare the patient, its primary purpose was to prepare the *ambulatory surgery unit* to receive and care for the patient in the most effective and efficient manner. If this occurred, the patient was more likely to progress through the other phases of care without unnecessary delays or surprises. This realization of purpose, along with the understanding of the interconnectedness of operational and clinical processes (see the three core process model section in Chapter 4), played an important role in redesigning the patient-flow process.

Previous efforts to improve other surgery-related processes, such as the patient preregistration process, achieved just that—an improved preregistration process. An understanding of the purpose of the pre-admission phase of care led the surgery team to look at preregistration in a different way. The team identified an entire package of information required before a patient's admission that helped prepare the care providers and the facility to most efficiently provide the outpatient surgery. This package included not only registration information (e.g., patient demographics and insurance data), but also patient education materials, clinical preparation of the patient (e.g., laboratory results, special orders, and patient history), surgery scheduling, and information about the surgical procedure so that any special equipment or supplies could be arranged for in advance. A pre-admission information-gathering process was then designed to help assemble this package of information during a patient encounter at the physician's office and make sure the information package had arrived at the hospital in advance of the patient's admission. A phone call to the patient the day before surgery confirmed last-minute details and provided the patient with an opportunity to ask any additional questions. In this way, the facility and care providers were better prepared to receive the patient, provide individualized care, anticipate and prevent delays or cancellations as a result of miscommunication or lack of information, and decrease the preoperative length of stay (Kelly et al. 1997).

While this approach to ambulatory surgery is commonplace today, the example is included here to offer insight regarding the role of purpose (explicitly or intuitively) in shaping the contemporary standard of care.

Fostering Common Ground

Without a clear understanding of what has to be accomplished, discussions on alternative solutions to a problem often lead to an impasse. Selecting one approach over another is hindered because people often bring to the discussion their own intense ownership of a particular solution, intervention, or idea. Discussing purpose can be a less threatening way to begin a discussion about a problem. Rather than highlighting differences among possible options and inviting comments on their perceived merit or shortcomings, discussing purpose helps to create a common ground from which to focus people with divergent opinions and views.

For example, consider two executives living in Seattle scheduled to present a lecture together at a professional conference in Chicago. The executives' presentation is on Monday at 11:00 am. They must be back in Seattle by Wednesday at noon for a board of directors meeting. They are considering various travel options. The purpose is to get from Seattle to Chicago. They find numerous means of travel that will achieve this purpose. They may drive, take a train, or fly. They further refine the purpose to get from Seattle to Chicago and back to meet the Monday and Wednesday obligations. If one wants to drive and one wants to fly, this refined purpose now leaves only one option: to fly. Next, they must decide upon airlines, routes, etc. Rather than arguing over the options, they add decision criteria to guide their decision: they would like to fly nonstop within a specified price range and time of day. They find two flights on different airlines. Because they are frequent fliers on the same airlines, they easily choose the flight on their preferred airline. Even if the two executives start with different ideas about their travel, clarifying their purpose and adding decision criteria naturally lead them to a common decision.

Understanding purpose to foster common ground may be extended to the use of clinical decision support in health services organizations. Information systems are used for a variety of purposes: storing, retrieving, and streamlining and automating access to data. Many information systems began as accounting systems. As more clinical applications are being developed and demands for electronic medical records and computerized physician order entry increase, questioning the purpose of these systems is important to ensure that the purpose, applications, uses, and outcomes are all aligned.

Reviewing early efforts in designing electronic clinical-decision-support tools provides insights about the role of purpose in enhancing successful implementation of new technology. The clinical epidemiology and medical informatics team at LDS Hospital in Salt Lake City, Utah, has used computerized systems to improve patient care for more than 30 years. In 1998, an article in the *New England Journal of Medicine* described the development of LDS Hospital's computer-assisted management program for antibiotics and other anti-infective agents (Evans et al. 1998). (For more information on the details of the technology, see the reference list at the end of this book.) This is how the LDS Hospital's team defined the purpose of clinical information systems: "The project was designed to augment physicians' judgment, not to replace it. The computer was simply a tool that offered data on individual patients, decision logic, and prescribing information to physicians in a useful and non-threatening way" (Garibaldi 1998).

The purpose of the clinical information system was to support decision making, and this in turn promoted cooperation between information specialists and clinicians. A clear description of the purpose can create common ground for diverse members of a group, contribute to their ability to focus on a common goal, and enlist buy-in to enhance successful implementation of initiatives to improve patient outcomes.

Promoting Breakthrough Ideas and Solutions

Lessons from public health offer examples of innovative solutions within the context of understanding purpose. Three types of prevention exist (Merrill and Timmreck 2006, 16–17):

- **Primary prevention** is preventing a disease or disorder before it happens.
- **Secondary prevention** is aimed at health screening and detection activities [to] block the progression of disease.
- **Tertiary prevention** blocks the progression of a disability, condition, or disorder to keep it from advancing and requiring excessive care.

Consider the historical treatment of infectious diseases. Victims of smallpox were quarantined to prevent the disease from spreading. A more effective solution emerged when the scientific thinking about infectious disease changed from containing the disease to strengthening a person's defenses against a disease. This powerful redefinition of purpose ultimately led to the development of vaccines (Barquet and Domingo 1997). The magnitude of the innovation has been described this way: "Indeed, if you asked a public health professional to draw up a top-ten list of the achievements of the past century, he or she would be hard pressed not to rank immunization first. Millions of lives have been saved and microbes stopped in their tracks before they could have a chance to wreak havoc. In short, the vaccine represents the single greatest promise of biomedicine: disease prevention" (Stern and Markel 2005, 611–12).

The Purpose Principle

Managers must develop the habit of asking themselves, "What are we really trying to achieve? On the basis of changes in the environment, technology, or customer requirements, what is our purpose? Does our current method of operating serve that purpose, or are there more effective alternatives?" When the purpose is clear, new solutions usually become clear as well.

The **purpose principle** is a tool to aid managers in this process. It comes from the concept of breakthrough thinking (Nadler and Hibino 1994), an approach to problem solving developed from the study of effective leaders and problem solvers from various industries and disciplines. Nadler and Hibino (1994, 1) found that "when confronted with a problem,

Primary prevention preventing a disease or disorder before it happens (Merrill and Timmreck 2006, 16)

Secondary prevention activities "aimed at health screening and detection activities [to] block the progression of disease" (Merrill and Timmreck 2006, 17)

Tertiary prevention intervention that "blocks the progression of a disability, condition, or disorder to keep it from advancing and requiring excessive care" (Merrill and Timmreck 2006, 17)

Purpose principle a tool to aid managers in identifying the right purpose to address successful people tend to question why they should spend their time and effort solving the problem at all," and that effective problem solvers "always placed every problem into a larger context . . . to understand the relationship between what effective action on the problem was supposed to achieve and the purposes of the larger setting of which the original problem was a part." By questioning purpose and enlarging the boundaries from which they examined the problem, effective problem solvers are able to purposely and systematically choose the right problem and, in turn, the best solution.

Discussions of purpose encourage accompanying mental models regarding the problem and solution to be brought into the open. Purpose may be considered a systemic structure and the purpose principle a tool that promotes double-loop learning by challenging assumptions about the nature of a problem. By encouraging the viewing of the problem and solution from the larger context of the entire system, the purpose principle also promotes an understanding of the connections between the problem at hand and other elements or components of the system.

From Concept to Practice

A series of questions can help managers to examine and clarify purpose. The first question should be, "What am I trying to accomplish?" Sometimes the response to this question results in a directional statement (improve, reduce). It is important to remember that action verbs describe a purpose (provide, build) while directional verbs describe a goal. To focus on the purpose rather than a goal, ask next: "What is this process, intervention, or department designed to accomplish?"

The purpose principle continues with a series of questions to expand the purpose. Unlike the 5 Why's tool of Lean to reduce the problem to a lesser problem or a root cause (ASQ 2010a), the purpose principle is used to identify and understand how the problem is related to the larger context in which it exists. Think of an onion. The effort of expanding the purpose is like starting from the inside of an onion and adding on the layers to construct a whole onion rather than peeling the onion, which is typically how the onion metaphor is presented. In this way, the larger purposes may be identified—and more layers are added to the onion. When the original purpose has been expanded several times, then another question should be asked: "What larger purpose might eliminate the need to achieve this smaller purpose?" (Nadler and Hibino 1994, 154).

Example 1

Here is an example to illustrate how the purpose principle might be used. The CEO of a large, tertiary care hospital closely follows his hospital's performance on the Hospital Quality Alliance (HQA) Performance Indicators and compares his organization's performance with that of the other hospitals in the community, in the state, and across the nation using the Hospital

Compare website. Although his hospital has shown steady improvement in the original indicators of congestive heart failure (CHF), community-acquired pneumonia (CAP), and acute myocardial infarction (AMI) over the past several years, the percentile rankings are disappointing, as other hospitals are also steadily improving in these three areas. He wonders why the CAP indicators are still showing results well below AMI and CHF and why the hospital shows three different results in the smoking cessation indicator (the one indicator common to all three conditions). He also wonders why the hospital is not doing as well in the more recently added indicators. The CEO ponders the series of purpose questions to redefine the organization's quality goals.

- *What am I trying to accomplish?*
  Improve my hospital's performance in the CMS quality indicators.
- *What is the process I am investigating? (note: defining the process/ activities helps to shift one's response from the directional verb "improve" to an action verb representing the purpose)*
  Measuring and reporting performance indicators on selected diseases as required by CMS.
- *Have I further expanded the purpose? What is the purpose of measuring and reporting performance indicators?*
  Performance indicators provide feedback about how we are doing as an organization. In our case, this feedback could suggest:
  o we provide quality care and my organization just doesn't docu-ment what we do very well;
  o we have many different ways of doing the same thing; and
  o because the CMS indicators are evidence-based (i.e., specific indi-cators represent actions shown by scientific studies to improve the quality of outcomes for that disease), our clinical protocols may not be based on the most current evidence; come to think of it, I wonder if we have clinical protocols . . . ?
- *Have I further expanded the purpose? What is the purpose of perfor-mance feedback?*
  Feedback in a complex organization provides information about the behavior of the system; from this feedback, I am beginning to real-ize that the organization is operating like a lot of little systems: indi-vidual physicians making their own decisions, individual departments involved in their own improvement efforts; individual diseases as the focus of clinical management.
- *Have I further expanded the purpose? What is the purpose of providing information about the behavior of the system?*
  The purpose of providing information about the behavior of the system is to better understand the system. If we don't understand the system, we won't be able to improve it. If we don't change the

behavior of the system, we are only treating symptoms of the problem. We need to be able to change to function more cooperatively as a system.

- *For the patients, what is the purpose?*

  Reporting quality indicators gives patients quality information to allow them to choose providers; however, employers and insurance companies will use the information more than patients.

- *For clinical staff, what is the purpose?*

  Clinical staff may see these quality indicators as just "one more thing to do" or as a hassle. They may not realize that these indicators actually reflect evidence-based practice or that performance on these indicators may eventually determine reimbursement.

- *What larger purpose may eliminate the need to achieve this smaller purpose altogether?*

  Going back to the "old days," when all these groups like CMS and The Joint Commission weren't telling us what to do to the extent they are today.

- *What is the right purpose for me to be working on? Describe how this purpose differs or does not differ from my original purpose.*

  CMS performance indicators may be used to promote improvement for the organization *overall*, which is different from what I was originally trying to achieve: improve my hospital's performance on the CMS quality indicators. If I look at the indicators as feedback about our system, I realize my purpose is to listen to the feedback to better understand the system.

- *Review my responses to the questions above. Given my understanding of purpose, what quality goals will I now set?*

  ○ Coordinate and align improvement efforts throughout the organization.

  ○ Evaluate and improve the process for identifying stakeholder requirements and integrating them into how we conduct business.

  ○ Identify and improve system processes, such as patient discharge and teaching; updating current evidence and incorporating it into how we treat patients; and performance data collection, analysis, and review.

Example 2

Here is another example of how the purpose might be used. The administrator for a large, multispecialty, ambulatory medical practice has implemented a new performance management system for the entire organization. When the office manager for one of the obstetrics and gynecology (OB/GYN) practices is given the first "clinic report card," the data show that, for obstetrics patients, the practice has performed well in the area of pregnancy-associated complications. However, the practice has performed poorly in the areas of patient satisfaction. In particular, patients are not satisfied with their level of involvement in their own care and their preparation for labor, delivery, breast-feeding, and care of their newborns.

The manager knows staff members are committed to quality patient care and are hard workers. Out of curiosity, the manager asks one of the obstetricians, "What is the purpose of prenatal care and the prenatal office visits?" The physician replies, "To identify signs of problems with the mother or the fetus and to intervene early to prevent problems from getting worse." The manager then asks the physician what kinds of problems could potentially occur, to which he replies, "Conditions like toxemia in the mother or growth retardation in the fetus."

The manager initially identifies the problem as patient dissatisfaction with prenatal care; the process to be improved as prenatal care; and the purpose of the prenatal visits (as described by the physician) as early identification of and intervention with problems with the mother and the fetus or baby. The manager then asks a series of purpose questions:

- *What am I trying to accomplish?*
  To improve the clinic's "report card" results in the area of patient dissatisfaction with prenatal care.
- *Have I expanded the purposes of addressing this problem? What is the purpose of the clinic's "report card"?*
  To monitor patient satisfaction with the care they receive in our clinic.
- *Have I further expanded the purpose? What is the purpose of monitoring patient satisfaction with the care they receive in our clinic?*
  To keep existing patients and to attract new patients to our clinic.
- *Have I further expanded the purpose? What is the purpose of keeping existing patients and attracting new patients to our clinic?*
  To stay in business and pay the bills.
- *For physicians, what is the purpose of prenatal care?*
  To identify signs of problems with the mother or the fetus and to intervene early to prevent problems from getting worse.
- *For patients, what is the purpose of prenatal care?*
  To have a healthy pregnancy and a healthy baby. To learn about prenatal classes and other parenting resources.
- *For the insurance companies, what is the purpose of prenatal care?*
  To prevent complications that require extended hospitalization of the mother or the baby and to keep overall healthcare costs down.
- *What larger purpose would eliminate the need to achieve these smaller purposes altogether?*
  If nobody got pregnant or had babies.

- *What is the right purpose for me to be working on? How does this purpose differ or not differ from my original purpose?*

  By answering these questions, it becomes apparent that the physicians, the office manager, the patients, and the insurance companies have somewhat different yet overlapping purposes. The purpose principle may be used to align all of these parties around a common purpose. A more comprehensive purpose for prenatal care that addresses all of the stakeholder requirements/purposes would be more effective.

  For example: The purpose of the clinic's prenatal services is to assess, monitor, and manage the physiological and psychosocial needs of families during the childbearing process.

By questioning, identifying, and documenting different purposes, the manager or team may select the most appropriate level of purpose, which is the purpose that enables them to solve the right problem and that is within their means (e.g., resources, scope of authority). At first the questions may be difficult to answer and may appear to be redundant. However, like anything new, with practice the ability to answer the questions will improve, and the repetition will encourage a deeper level of thinking about the problem.

Improving System Performances: Corollaries to Purpose

Once the purpose is defined, the activities to achieve that purpose may be defined according to the different stakeholders. Clarifying corollaries to the purpose may be helpful to ensure that the various stakeholders or discussion participants can see that their ideas are addressed.

For the OB/GYN clinic described above, examples of such corollaries include the following:

- The desired *results* are healthy clinical outcomes, satisfied patients, and cost-effective services.
- The clinic will *measure* how successful it is in achieving the desired results with the following data: maternal and infant complication rates, early diagnosis, patient satisfaction, payer satisfaction, and so on.
- The *service mix, processes,* and *interventions* used to accomplish the purpose may then be strategically determined, designed, and improved.
- The *goals* for performance improvement efforts may be to validate the purposes of the key stakeholders identified earlier; refine the clinic's purpose for prenatal care services based on any new information obtained; evaluate current practices to determine the extent to which the clinic is accomplishing its purpose; define a service mix that is consistent with the purpose; prioritize those services needing

improvement; and design, redesign, and implement improved processes that meet all stakeholder requirements and accomplish the new definition of purpose.

Although the results of this example may seem intuitive or obvious, without the discussion of purpose, the clinic manager may set goals to improve the esthetics surrounding care, rather than the actual care processes themselves.

Vision

In the examples, the desired results may also be considered the ideal future state or **vision** for the practice. Vision plays a role in leadership (Kouzes and Posner 2007), personal effectiveness (Covey 2004), organizational effectiveness (Senge 2006), art (Fritz 1989), and even survival (Frankl 1962).

Vision
ideal future state

Vision and purpose go hand in hand. Purpose represents the identity; vision represents this identity in its ideal future state. Visions may be found at a variety of levels within health services. For example, the Healthy People initiative, coordinated by the Office of Disease Prevention and Health Promotion within the US Department of Health and Human Services, offers an overall vision for the nation's health: "A society in which all people live long, healthy lives" (Healthy People 2011). This vision provides a common direction for diverse groups that share the interest of improving health and healthcare within the United States so they may individualize their own community visions within the larger national context. As shown in Exhibit 5.1, the Healthy People vision is complemented with the corollaries to purpose described previously. The future desired state (results) is represented in the vision and overarching goals; the purpose of the Healthy People 2020 initiative is represented by the mission; the services, processes, and categories of interventions used to accomplish the purpose are identified accordingly in the defined priority topic areas; the improvement goals are represented by the objectives within these topics; and the measures of success are represented by the health indicators within four major categories.

Organizations often have an overall vision for the future. Managers may also use the concept of vision in a variety of ways and at various levels within the organization. Managers may have visions for their careers, for their own professional contribution to quality healthcare, or for their ideal departments or service areas. Managers may ask a team to describe its ideal vision for a particular work process or process of care. In creating a vision, describing ideal characteristics rather than ideal interventions allows flexibility in how the vision will be accomplished while fostering adaptability to changing internal and external conditions. For example, questions that physicians may pose when creating a vision for their own office practice include the following list.

EXHIBIT 5.1

Healthy People 2020

Vision and Overarching Goals of Healthy People 2020	

A society in which all people live long, healthy lives.

- Attain high-quality, longer lives free of preventable disease, disability, injury, and premature death
- Achieve health equity, eliminate disparities, and improve the health of all groups
- Create social and physical environments that promote good health for all
- Promote quality of life, healthy development, and healthy behaviors across all life stages

Mission of Healthy People 2020

- Identify nationwide health improvement priorities
- Increase public awareness and understanding of the determinants of health, disease, and disability and the opportunities for progress
- Provide measurable objectives and goals that are applicable at the national, state, and local levels
- Engage multiple sectors to take actions to strengthen policies and improve practices that are driven by the best available evidence and knowledge
- Identify critical research, evaluation, and data collection needs

Topics

Examples of topics and an example of recommended intervention(s)

- Adolescent health: therapeutic foster care
- Cancer: screen for breast, cervical, colorectal cancer
- Environmental safety: test older homes for presence of lead paint
- Heart disease and stroke: Worksite nutrition and physical activity programs
- Immunizations and infectious diseases: targeted vaccinations
- Mental health and mental disorders: screening for depression in adults
- Nutrition and weight status: screening for obesity in children and adolescence
- Substance abuse: community interventions to reduce alcohol impaired driving

Objectives

Examples of objectives:

- Reduce the annual number of new cases of diagnosed diabetes in the population

(*continued*)

- Increase the proportion of persons with health insurance

EXHIBIT 5.1

- Reduce infections caused by key pathogens transmitted commonly through food
- Increase the proportion of women with a family history of breast and/or ovarian cancer who receive genetic counseling
- Reduce the number of new AIDS cases among adolescents and adults
- Increase access to trauma care in the United States

Categories of Measures

- General health status
- Determinants of health
- Health-related quality of life and well-being
- Disparities

Source: Healthy People (2011).

If my practice were recognized as one of the best in the country,

- What would patients and families say about the care they received?
- What would patients and families say about their interactions with me? With my office staff?
- What would my colleagues around the country say about my practice?
- What processes in my office would colleagues most want to emulate?

In addition, physicians may want to consider these questions:

- How do I and my office staff feel after a day's work?
- If a prominent journal or newspaper were writing about my office practice, what would the article say?

When creating a vision, one should not be limited by what is possible or what is not possible. By defining characteristics of the ideal future rather than ideal interventions, a manager may balance describing an ideal future with present constraints. When asked about their ideal unit or office, healthcare workers often respond with, "We would have that new computer system" or "We would totally remodel the office." However, financial constraints may not allow for these expenditures, which makes constructing the vision an exercise in futility rather than a chance to describe a future ideal state. Rather than "We would have that new computer system," the ideal answer might be, "We have streamlined, user-friendly documentation and communication mechanisms in place to provide needed information for safe care, efficient internal office operations, and patient education." Rather than "We would totally remodel the office," the ideal answer might be, "Patients will find a clean, accessible, comfortable, and relaxing office environment that respects their privacy and confidentiality."

By defining characteristics of the ideal future rather than ideal interventions, opportunities for finding creative and flexible ways of achieving the vision while working within the constraints of the situation may be enhanced.

Context

Context

"the unquestioning assumptions through which all experience is filtered" (Davis 1982, 26)

In Chapter 3, the concept of mental models is introduced as a deeply ingrained way of thinking that influences how a person sees and understands the world and how a person acts. **Context** is a concept closely related to mental models and is defined as "the unquestioning assumptions through which all experience is filtered" (Davis 1982). In this book, the phrase "mental models" refers to an individual's assumptions, and the term "context" refers to organizational assumptions that guide how the organization defines itself and how it operates.

The following two examples illustrate the subtle difference between mental models and context. Here is the first illustration.

> Consider this analogy. You inherit your grandmother's house. Unknown to you is one peculiarity: all the light fixtures have bulbs that give off a blue rather than yellow light. You find that you don't like the feel of the rooms and spend a lot of time and money repainting walls, reupholstering furniture, and replacing carpets. You never seem to get it quite right, but nonetheless, you rationalize that at least it is improving with each thing you do. Then one day you notice the blue light bulbs and change them. Suddenly, all that you fixed is broken.
>
> Context is like the color of the light, not the objects in the room. Context colors everything in the corporation. More accurately, the context alters what we see, usually without our being aware of it. (Goss, Pascale, and Athos 1998, 88–89)

High-reliability organizations (HROs)

"organizations with systems in place that are exceptionally consistent in accomplishing their goals and avoiding potentially catastrophic errors" (AHRQ 2008b)

An external community focus may represent one operating context for a health services organization, while an internal organizational focus may represent a different operating context. A focus on improving the quality of health services delivered may represent one operating context, while a focus on improving health of the community is another. Management decisions about resource allocation, prevention, or continuum-of-care issues differ depending on the context or assumptions about the organization's focus or role in the community.

An emerging context for health services organizations is the **high-reliability organization** (HRO), defined as "organizations with systems in place that are exceptionally consistent in accomplishing their goals and avoiding potentially catastrophic errors" (AHRQ 2008b). Complementing the perspective of human error (Chapter 4), HROs "emphasize a way of thinking about issues" (AHRQ 2008b). Within an HRO context, all individuals are encouraged to actively look for interdependencies within the system and to aggressively seek to know what they don't know (Roberts and Bea 2001). An HRO context influences managerial functions as managers in HROs "design reward and incentive systems to recognize costs of failures as well as benefits of reliability . . . [and] consistently communicate the big picture of what the organization seeks to do and try to get everyone to communicate with others about how they fit in the big picture" (Roberts and Bea 2001, 71).

Consider this second illustration of context, which suggests a corollary to the concept: content.

> Most parents have dreams for their children. Some want their children to be doctors, some musicians, and all want them to be healthy, wealthy, and wise. These are parents raising their children by focusing on content. Following in a father's footsteps, or in the footsteps father never had and therefore wants for his son, [is a] well-known example of this approach. Other parents, however, raise their children by focusing on context. In Helen Keller's famous phrase, their dream is, "be all you can be." The orientation here is to "parent" the context and let the child discover the content. (Davis 1982, 28)

As stated in the illustration, managers may also find themselves facing the dichotomy of which to manage: context or content. One may think of the distinctions between context and content as they are illustrated by a circle. The boundary of the circle is the context; the inside of the circle is the content (Davis 1982). Historically, health services managers have been promoted on the basis of their content expertise: an excellent pharmacist becomes the manager of the entire pharmacy department; an excellent engineer becomes the manager of the facilities maintenance department; or an excellent clinician becomes a department, division, or unit manager. These managerial roles generally include direct supervision of the people and the work.

Today, the organizations, environments, processes, and technologies in the health services industry are so complex that managers cannot be experts on both managing and on the content of the work that needs to be managed. Managers' roles will increasingly move away from managing content to managing context. This means employees with fundamental knowledge of the work itself will carry out and improve their work processes, while managers will ensure that employees have the appropriate tools, information, knowledge, and competency to effectively do their jobs and deliver quality services and products.

Managing context also suggests managing the boundaries of the system, which may be a unit, a department, an office practice, a service line, or an entire organization. Boundaries may be defined in terms of scope of work, decision-making authority, expectations, and accountability. The manager may set or reset the boundaries on the basis of environmental conditions and other organizational considerations. In a department with a high ratio of experienced employees, the manager may expand the boundary so that staff are more autonomous in their decision making. However, in a department composed of a young or inexperienced staff, the manager may tighten the boundaries of decision making until the employees gain knowledge, ability, and confidence in their own decision-making skills.

Managing the boundaries of the system also suggests that the managers define not only their own areas of responsibility but also the interfaces that occur at the boundaries. As healthcare organizations become more complex and teams are increasingly used to accomplish the organization's work, the supervisory role also shifts to one of "boundary manager" (Fisher 2000). This means that, rather than supervising individuals, the supervisor helps teams interact with each other to coordinate work, communicate information, or resolve problems. Likewise, effectively managing context requires an awareness and understanding of the interfaces with other systems within and outside of the organization. In the trade-offs example described in Chapter 2, the manager who anticipated unintended consequences of reducing hospital length of stay and proactively worked with the nursing homes demonstrated an awareness and understanding of the interface between acute care and nursing home care.

The best way to become aware of context and draw the appropriate boundary for the system is by asking the right questions (Davis 1982). For managers, the key to asking the right questions is to be willing to challenge current assumptions; otherwise, the answers to the questions will simply be restatements of what is already known, and the questioning process will not help the manager understand and explore what is beyond the current boundary of knowledge or awareness.

The importance of challenging assumptions (e.g., double-loop learning) may be seen in the ambulatory surgery improvement example in Chapter 4. The prevailing assumption at the time was to use restructuring to reduce costs, specifically, to reduce the number of registered nurse (RN) positions by eliminating RNs or replacing them with unlicensed personnel (Gordon 2005). In the ambulatory surgery example, "because the outcome of cost savings and value had been defined at the onset of the project in terms of length of stay and total consumption of resources, not just in terms of staffing mix, cost savings [were] realized despite a predominantly RN staff" (Kelly et al. 1997, 126). By questioning the assumption that restructuring was the only solution and replacing it with a principles-driven change process, this team was able to improve throughput, reduce costs, maintain clinical outcomes, and improve patient satisfaction while retaining RNs in their care-delivery model. This approach was "quite different from the trend of decreasing professional staff and increasing mix of unlicensed support personnel" (Kelly et al. 1997, 128).

Summary

Understanding the role of mission, vision, and context as underlying structures is essential for managers to continuously adapt and improve in the presence of complexity and uncertainty. The mission or purpose describes the identity of the organization—the reason it exists. Within this identity, the vision (the ideal future state) and context are defined.

The purpose principle aids in clarifying, defining, or validating purpose. The relationship between vision and context is illustrated with the example of a young child putting together a puzzle. The child empties the puzzle pieces from the box and props up the box to see a picture of what the puzzle is supposed to look like when it is completed. He then sorts the pieces: one group contains pieces with a straight edge or a corner shape, and one group contains the odd shapes. When asked why, the child replies, "To make the outside first." Once the outer edge of the puzzle is assembled, he goes about fitting in the rest of the pieces, knowing that each piece will eventually have its own place in the picture.

The manager's role in establishing vision may be thought of as making sure everyone in the organization has the ability to see the entire picture—that is, what the puzzle will look like when it is completed. The manager's role in setting the boundaries or context of the system may be thought of as putting together the outer edge of the puzzle. The images or shapes of the individual pieces may be thought of as the content, which is what goes on or what is done within the organization. Although there is much ambiguity at first about where the individual pieces should go, enough information is available to continue the task of building the puzzle, or, in the manager's case, moving toward the vision of the future.

Exercise

Objectives: To think about and clarify professional purpose.

Instructions:
- Write your own professional purpose or mission.
- Practice the purpose principle by writing your responses to the following questions as they relate to your professional purpose:
  a. What am I trying to accomplish?
  b. What is the process(es) or activity(ies) involved in the response to a? (Be sure to use an active, not directional, verb.)
  c. What is the purpose of the response to b?
  d. What is the purpose of the response to c?
  e. What is the purpose of the response to d?
  f. What is my purpose according to my patients/clients/customers?
  g. What larger purpose may eliminate the need to achieve this smaller purpose altogether?

h. What is the right purpose for me to be working on? Describe how this purpose differs or does not differ from my original purpose.

Companion Readings

Gary, L. 2003. "What High-Reliability Organizations Know." *Harvard Management Update*, December, 3–5.

Nadler, G., and W. J. Chandon. 2004. "Introducing the Smart Question Approach: Moving Beyond Problem-Solving to Creating Solutions." In *Smart Questions: Learn to Ask the Right Questions for Powerful Results*, 1–41. San Francisco: Jossey-Bass.

Shuman, J., and J. Twombly. 2010. "Collaborative Networks Are the Organization: An Innovation in Organization Design and Management." *Vikalpa: The Journal for Decision Makers* 35 (1): 1–13.

Web Resources

Agency for Healthcare Research and Quality. 2008. *Becoming a High Reliability Organization: Operational Advice for Hospital Leaders.* www.ahrq.gov/qual/hroadvice/

Agency for Healthcare Research and Quality: "Surveys on Patient Safety Culture" www.ahrq.gov/qual/patientsafetyculture/

ESTABLISHING IMPROVEMENT GOALS IN COMPLEX SYSTEMS

Learning Objectives

After completing this chapter you should be able to:

- appreciate the impact of setting goals in complex systems;
- identify various mental models about goals;
- link improvement goal statements with the ability to achieve desired improvement results; and
- differentiate advantages and disadvantages of different types of goal statements.

Patient A presents to his primary care provider as overweight and suffering from high blood pressure. The treatment goals the provider sets for the patient are to lose weight and to take the prescribed blood pressure medicine. The patient begins dieting and taking his blood pressure medicine. Within six months, Patient A has lost 30 pounds and shows improved blood pressure. However, at Patient A's annual checkup several months later, his provider is dismayed to find that he has gained back the 30 pounds.

Patient B is also overweight and suffering from high blood pressure when she sees her primary care provider. The treatment goals the provider sets for the patient are to integrate a balanced diet and regular exercise into her daily lifestyle and to reduce blood pressure through lifestyle change and medication. Within six months, Patient B has also lost 30 pounds and shows improved blood pressure. At her next annual physical, Patient B has kept off the 30 pounds and informs her provider that she feels much better as she has been walking three days a week and eating healthier.

The seemingly subtle difference in how the treatment goals were set for these two patients actually represents the relationship between the goals and the subsequent results that are obtained.

Goals serve a variety of purposes for individuals throughout the realm of health services. Clinical providers use goals when establishing plans of care, not just in primary care as in the previous example, but in all settings. For example, goals may be set for managing a patient's respiratory status in an intensive care unit, targeting functional activity in the rehabilitation setting, planning a patient's discharge from a hospital, and promoting comfort and end-of-life care in palliative and hospice services. Managers use goals when conducting employee performance appraisals to determine how well employees are fulfilling their job responsibilities, to target areas for improvement, and to guide rewards and incentives. Project managers use goals when implementing administrative and clinical information systems. Goals inform every step of the project management process and are the bases for timelines focused on capital purchases, information system programming needs, capital purchases, user training, and installation. Faculty use goals (also referred to as learning objectives) when teaching health services professionals. Health educators use goals when designing health prevention and promotion programs targeting smoking, obesity, and hypertension. Program managers and researchers use goals when writing grant proposals.

Goals also serve a variety of purposes when considered from the organizational level (Scott 2003). Strategic goals are used to provide direction for decision making. An organizational goal to increase market share in obstetrics influences management decisions about prioritizing capital expenditures for remodeling patient care units in the hospital. Organizational goals, such as being the first-choice medical provider in the community, may serve to motivate employees and other stakeholders. A goal to become a "center of excellence" for cardiovascular care may foster employee pride and loyalty, serve as a recruitment strategy for physicians and other clinical providers, and bring prestige within the community. A goal to be the "premiere center for cancer research" can legitimize investment in research infrastructure at an academic medical center; successful research, in turn, will position the center to acquire additional research funding.

An organization's effectiveness in setting and aligning goals gives one clues about its path along the quality continuum. Exhibit 1.3 illustrates how the quality continuum may be viewed when considering its focus on products, processes, customers, and costs of poor quality. The Baldrige Performance Excellence Program systems model (Chapter 4) offers a systems view

EXHIBIT 6.1

Goals and the Quality Continuum

| Reacting to problems: strategic and operational *goals* are poorly defined | Early systemic approach: strategic and quantitative *goals* are beginning to be defined | Aligned approach: processes address key strategies and *goals* of the organization | Integrated approach: processes and measures track progress on key strategic and operational *goals* |

Less mature ——————————————————————————→ More mature

Source: National Institute of Standards and Technology (2011, 66).

on the quality continuum, which includes the role of goals and is illustrated in Exhibit 6.1 (NIST 2011, 66; Kelly 2009a).

When one realizes how pervasively goals are used by individuals and organizations within clinical and non-clinical settings, one may begin to appreciate the widespread impact of effective goal-setting skills on organizational performance. The importance of setting effective goals may be further appreciated when one realizes that all subsequent actions follow and are influenced by how the initial goal is set.

Relationship Between Goals and Results

A guest lecturer, formerly a neonatal intensive care nurse, leads health administration doctoral students in a discussion about organizational effectiveness. At the conclusion of the discussion, one student observes that the previous guest lecturer also had a background in pediatrics. The student asks if there is a relationship between an interest in quality and a background in pediatrics. The guest lecturer replies, "Maybe it's because we see life at its beginning and understand how important a healthy start to life is."

The ability to set goals effectively is a requisite skill for managers at all levels of an organization. The following example of two hospitals facing a similar challenge illustrates how goals set by leadership influence subsequent actions and the results of those actions.

The Hospital Consumer Assessment of Healthcare Providers and Systems (HCAHPS) reports for Hospital A and Hospital B show that both perform below the national average for hospitals of a similar size and type. Senior leaders at each hospital decide to focus on improving customer service and patient satisfaction as an organizational priority. To address the problem of low patient satisfaction, the senior management team at Hospital A sets the following goal: improve customer service.

To achieve this goal, Hospital A hires a customer service specialist and institutes mandatory customer service training for all employees. The nurse managers in the hospital are faced with a dilemma. Their department education budgets are limited, and their staff are already subject to mandatory education in areas such as infection control and fire safety. One more mandatory educational requirement will deplete the education dollars and eliminate the managers' resources for funding continuing education to maintain the staff's clinical competence.

Hospital B uses a different approach to address the problem of low patient satisfaction. Because the source of the problem was not evident to Hospital B's administrators, they first try to gain a better understanding of why the problem is occurring. The senior management team at Hospital B sets the following partial or intermediate goal: understand why patients are not satisfied with their hospital experience. This goal guides further study of the hospital's satisfaction data, which show that patients are least satisfied with the communication with nurses and feel rushed to leave the hospital without being fully prepared to do so. The organization conducts a root-cause analysis to learn why communication and discharge planning are not occurring effectively. The analysis reveals that, although staffing seems adequate on a day-to-day basis, the hospital's reliance on temporary staff and traveling nurses has increased significantly over the past year. Although the temporary staff and traveling nurses are experienced in their technical duties, their lack of familiarity with the hospital's specific procedures and resources increasingly leads to communication breakdowns within and among departments. The organizational analysis highlights this common problem for the departments responsible for patient registration, billing, and housekeeping and in the nursing, respiratory therapy, and pharmacy departments. On the basis of this information, senior leaders at Hospital B prioritize the contributing factors and develop specific goals to address the top-priority factors. They revise their goals as follows: (1) increase the proportion of staff who are permanent employees, (2) improve the discharge planning process, (3) reallocate resources spent on temporary staff to fund the aforementioned improvements, and (4) monitor the impact of staffing and process improvements on patient satisfaction.

Repair service behavior
a type of problem solving where organizations or individuals solve a problem they know how to solve, whether or not it is the problem they need to solve (Dorner 1996)

Which hospital's goals are most likely to improve patients' satisfaction with their hospital experience? A vague goal offering little direction, like Hospital A's goal to "improve customer service," often results in the problem-solving approach called **repair service behavior**. Organizations or individuals are using repair service behavior when they solve a "problem" they know how to solve, whether or not it is the problem they need to solve (Dorner 1996). An example of repair service behavior is when a novice gardener responds to the problem of withering leaves on a new plant by watering more instead of repotting and fertilizing the plant, which is what the plant needs. Examples of repair service behavior in health services organizations can include creating new positions, conducting training, writing a new policy, or requesting more funds.

Hospital A knew how to create new positions and conduct training. However, it did not know how to identify the underlying cause of a widespread organizational problem. This example also illustrates how a poorly conceived goal (improve customer service) is likely to cause unintended consequences or create more problems in other areas of the organization. In this case, the mandatory customer-service training took resources away from technical education and over time risked reducing the overall technical competency of the nursing staff.

In contrast, Hospital B's response illustrates the senior leaders' understanding of how goal setting should be approached in complex systems such as healthcare organizations (Dorner 1996, 63–64).

- When working with a complex, dynamic system, first develop at least a *provisional picture of the partial goals to achieve*; those partial goals will clarify what needs to be done when.

- In complex situations, almost always avoid focusing on just one element and pursuing only one goal; instead, *pursue several goals at once.*

By approaching the problem using a partial goal (understand why patients are not satisfied with their hospital experience), Hospital B defined the underlying problems and then set the clear, multidimensional statement to guide the improvement interventions. Hospital B avoided an intervention that may not have solved the problem and was able to avoid the repair service behavior often associated with an unclear goal.

Though it is a requisite skill for managers, goal setting is an area where managers err. Several of the errors defined in *Management Mistakes in Healthcare* (Hofmann 2005, 11) are related to faulty goal setting within an organization's management or administrative domain. These errors include:

- inadequate preparation of/by decision maker(s);
- political pressure;
- a flawed decision-making process; and
- ignorance of legitimate alternatives.

By improving their goal-setting skills, managers not only promote positive movement along the quality continuum but also may decrease their contribution to latent management errors and, in turn, improve patient safety in their organizations.

Setting Improvement Goals in Complex Systems

Just as experience can influence how one defines "quality" (see Chapter 1), one's experience can influence one's mental models about setting goals. In some contexts, the SMART approach (a mnemonic for specific, measureable, achievable, realistic/relevant, timely) to setting goals is recommended. In some contexts, the accepted approach to goal setting is based on the definition of a goal as (Gitlin and Lyons 2008, 89):

> a clear and concise statement that represents what will be accomplished as a result of the program. It is a global or broad statement describing the overarching purpose(s) of the project or what will be achieved by conducting the proposed program. . . . In turn, each goal has a specific set of objectives. An objective is a statement about a specific outcome of a program that can be evaluated and measured. Thus, an objective must be written in such a way as to reflect a qualitative or quantitative measurement strategy.

This section is not intended to replace these and other approaches to planning. Rather, this section provides an alternative mental model regarding goals within the context of complex systems. Chapter 5 discusses how, by questioning purpose and enlarging the boundaries from which they examine the problem, effective problem solvers are able to purposely and systematically choose the right problem and, in turn, the best solution. Likewise, questioning goals within the context of complex systems can better enable managers to purposely and systematically choose goals that will help improve organizational performance and achieve desired results.

Use Intermediate Goals to Better Understand the Problem

Although vague, general, or unclear goals may lead to repair service behavior, phrasing a partial goal in general terms is useful to set the overall direction (as illustrated in the example of Hospital B). Specific goals can be established once decision makers gain new information and clarity about the problem. For example, a surgical services manager may use general goals to set the overall direction for his department over the next several years. These goals may be to improve clinical outcomes, improve patient satisfaction, improve cost effectiveness, and integrate services across multiple sites. Each year, during the annual planning process, specific short-term or intermediate goals may also be established. The goal in year 1 may be to implement a standard performance measurement system across all sites. The goal in year 2 may be to increase the percentage of first surgical cases for the day that are started on time for each of the operating rooms in the service. The goal in year 3 may be to implement standard preoperative testing protocols to eliminate unnecessary variation in preoperative tests (Kelly et al. 1997).

In this example, a general goal is used to communicate overall direction. Because the manager also understands the concept and importance of partial goals, he is able to establish the first partial goal (measurement system) to help him understand how to prioritize subsequent annual improvement goals.

Be Aware of Implicit Goals

An administrator with responsibility for a large community hospital's emergency department (ED) was challenged with delays and bottlenecks in transferring patients from the ED to inpatient beds. The administrator gave this improvement goal to the ED manager: decrease the time from decision to admit to the actual admission to 20 minutes or less. The improvement team organized to meet this goal found that one cause of delays was the numerous phone calls made to the receiving inpatient unit to coordinate the transfer with the nursing staff. The team decided upon this intervention: if by the third phone call the nurse was not available to receive a report on the patient by phone, the patient would be taken to the assigned room by the ED technician and the report faxed to the inpatient unit.

The team implemented the new process and the time to transfer dropped to 20 minutes or less. The implicit goal that was *not* conveyed by the administrator was to ensure that improvements were based on safe practices. Without this implicit goal being defined, the team became so focused on the

20-minute goal that their judgment of safe communications during handoffs was clouded. As a result, their "improvement" was in direct opposition to the National Patient Safety Goal "improve the effectiveness of communication among caregivers" (The Joint Commission 2010d).

An undefined implicit goal can contribute to a situation of accidental adversaries (see Chapter 3). In this ED example, such was the case between the manager and the administrator (the ED manager thought she was meeting her boss's goal while the administrator was dissatisfied with the team's efforts) and between the ED nurses and the inpatient nurses (each "blamed" the other for not understanding their patient flow–related issues).

In contrast, the surgical services manager in the previous example understands the concept of implicit goals. For example, the manager knows that to achieve the desired level of performance, cultivating positive and collaborative relationships between physicians and administrators is essential. Though not on the written list of goals, positive relationships are reinforced at every staff meeting and a philosophy of collaboration guides the manager in designing the performance measurement system and improving first-case start times. As a result of the manager's implicit goal of building relationships in years 1 and 2, implementing a clinical standard of care can be accomplished more smoothly in year 3.

Refine, Revise, and Reformulate as Needed

Managers may find that setting goals is an iterative process; that is, as new information becomes available, they must be willing to evaluate previous goals and reformulate them as needed. For example, a nurse manager of a 30-bed, medical-surgical patient unit was charged with improving the overall performance of her unit. Because the unit was the major inpatient unit of a small community hospital, she was faced with a major overhaul rather than simply a single improvement. However, she realized that the goal of "overhaul performance" was too vague to identify specific interventions, expectations, and action plans for her staff.

The manager reformulated her original goal—"overhaul performance"—to more clearly establish the general direction of the performance improvement effort. Her new goals were to (1) promote teamwork, (2) promote continuity of care, (3) meet or exceed local and national standards of care, (4) integrate performance improvement into the daily work environment, (5) promote staff satisfaction, and (6) improve cost effectiveness.

Understanding dynamic complexity (see Chapter 2) encourages managers to reformulate goals as new information becomes available or the original situation changes. In such cases, managers should not consider the practice of reformulating goals as a sign of indecisiveness or weak managerial skills; rather they should consider it validation of their understanding of complex dynamic systems.

Use Multiple Goals to Recognize System Relationships

The nurse manager in the previous example demonstrated another important approach for setting effective goals. Because of the interrelationships among activities, processes, and other elements in healthcare organizations, focusing on multiple interrelated goals is necessary. Although a single goal may be useful for a simple process improvement, a systems perspective suggests the need for setting multiple goals that may be carried out concurrently or sequentially to take into account the interrelationships within the system. The systems models in Chapter 4 may guide managers in identifying areas for consideration when establishing multiple goals.

In this medical-surgical unit, the nurse manager assembled a team of charge nurses to work together intensively to help determine how to meet the unit's goals. After several meetings directed toward understanding the hospital's history, operating requirements, and environmental challenges; analyzing current processes; and identifying causes of performance gaps, the team discussed its ideal vision for the unit. They described their ideal unit according to desired clinical outcomes, the nature of their relationships with patients and families, teamwork, and business requirements. This vision became the unit's long-term goal.

The members of the team focused on multiple interdependent interventions to achieve their vision. Although they would not be able to implement multiple interventions all at once because of resource constraints, the team realized the importance of identifying, prioritizing, and establishing timelines to accomplish the specific goals within the general direction set by the manager. Some of the interventions (e.g., establishing a staff communication book and bulletin board) could be implemented immediately without much effort. Some of the goals (e.g., improving the way in which daily census and productivity were tracked, reported, communicated, and managed) would take more time to implement and were identified as short-term goals. Other goals (e.g., clarifying care-team roles, structure, and job descriptions) required more in-depth development and implementation considerations and were identified as medium-term goals.

The team converted an implicit goal to an explicit one by adding the following long-term goal: enhance the personal accountability of all staff. Clear goals provided the direction; a performance measurement system and a simple project-tracking report enabled the manager, the team, and the unit staff to track their progress toward their goals and their progress toward becoming their ideal unit.

Types of Goal Statements

Along with setting effective goals, managers must purposefully craft a goal statement that will best help them succeed in a given situation. For example, a manager has just learned that the immunization rates for the patients in his large pediatric practice are below both the state and national averages. He is faced with the problem of substandard immunization rates. How does he now communicate improvement goals to the practice in ways that will use the approaches just described?

Some types of goal statements have been introduced through the examples presented earlier in the chapter. The different types of goals may be thought of as pairs of opposites: positive or negative, general or specific, clear or unclear, simple or multiple, and implicit or explicit (Dorner 1996). Exhibit 6.2 provides a definition for each of these types and examples of how each may be used by the manager of the pediatric practice.

EXHIBIT 6.2

Examples of Types of Goals

Definition	Type of Goal	Example
Working toward a desired condition	Positive	Achieve immunization rates that are in the top 10 percent statewide.
Making an undesirable condition go away	Negative	Reduce the number of patients with incomplete immunizations.
Few criteria	General	Improve immunization rates.
Multiple criteria	Specific	Ensure all infants in the practice receive the appropriate vaccinations at ages 1 month, 2 months, 4 months, 6 months, 12 months, 15 months, 18 months, and 24 months according to the Centers for Disease Control and Prevention Recommended Childhood Immunization Schedule.
Difficult to determine if the goal has been met	Unclear	Work with the office staff to improve pediatric care.
Precise criteria permitting the evaluation of whether the goal is being met	Clear	Our clinic will select a team to enroll in the quality improvement collaborative offered by the State Pediatric Association from April through September. The team will design and implement processes to improve the clinic's compliance with the Recommended Childhood Immunization Schedule. The team will measure overall immunization rates on a quarterly basis. Results will be reported at staff meetings.

(continued)

EXHIBIT 6.2
(continued)

Definition	Type of Goal	Example
Single goal	Simple	Give age-appropriate immunizations at each well-child appointment.
Series of sequential or concurrent goals that take into account relationships within the system	Multiple	Track patient compliance with well-child exams. Notify and schedule patients who have missed well-child exams. Give age-appropriate immunizations during well-child exams.
Hidden	Implicit (unstated)	Improve immunization rates.
Obvious	Explicit	Improve the ability to identify, deliver, and monitor pediatric preventive care services, including age-appropriate immunizations.

Source: Adapted from Dorner, D. 1996. *The Logic of Failure: Recognizing and Avoiding Error in Complex Situations.* Reading, MA: Perseus Books. Used with permission.

Critiquing Goal Statements

Goal statements need to be effective. When faced with a problem to solve, a manager may state the goal in different ways and evaluate the pros and cons of each statement as a way to enhance his decision-making skills. The goals in Exhibit 6.2 are critiqued here, listed in order of effectiveness, beginning with the most effective goal statement for the situation and ending with the least effective.

Explicit Goal: *Improve the ability to identify, deliver, and monitor pediatric preventive care services, including age-appropriate immunizations.*
    Of all the sample goals, the statement for the explicit goal is the most effective for the situation because it

- is appropriate for an improvement effort, not a daily operational expectation;
- addresses the underlying work processes linked to the desired clinical outcomes;
- incorporates changes in how the clinic functions as a whole, not just the individual encounter between the caregiver and the patient;
- includes an expectation for ongoing evaluation and continuous improvement;
- sets the stage for a highly leveraged intervention (by stating the goal in terms of preventive services and not simply immunizations, the

improved process will contribute to improvements in multiple results, not just a single outcome); and

- reflects an understanding of "upstream" processes that could influence results (identify preventive care services).

This goal statement actually is a combination of an explicit, a clear, a multiple, a specific, and a positive goal. As more experience is gained in setting goals, one will find that the most effective goals for an improvement effort usually contain a combination of all of these characteristics.

Clear Goal. *Our clinic will select a team to enroll in the quality improvement collaborative offered by the State Pediatric Association from April through September. The team will design and implement processes to improve the clinic's compliance with the Recommended Childhood Immunization Schedule. The team will measure overall immunization rates on a quarterly basis. Results will be reported at staff meetings.*

The clear goal is the next most effective goal statement for an effort to improve immunization rates in this scenario. This goal is also a combination statement, incorporating features of a clear, a multiple, a specific, and a positive goal. Although readers may like this goal because it is very clear, this goal statement includes the following pitfalls. First, because the focus is solely on immunizations, the opportunity to leverage this effort (i.e., the time and effort by the team) to influence a broader array of similar processes and services is lost. Although the broader scope may be implicit to the manager, the manager will likely get just what he asks for—an exclusive focus on immunizations. Second, the prescriptive nature of this goal statement may exclude opportunities for other possible and more effective solutions. By stating that results will be measured quarterly, the team may default to retrospective review and miss an opportunity to design a concurrent data collection process.

Specific Goal. *Ensure all infants in the practice receive the appropriate vaccinations at ages 1 month, 2 months, 4 months, 6 months, 12 months, 15 months, 18 months, and 24 months, according to the Centers for Disease Control and Prevention Recommended Childhood Immunization Schedule.*

Many readers will like this goal statement because it is very specific and, at first glance, appears to be an effective goal. However, this statement (similar to an objective as defined above) actually describes the results/data to be measured to determine if the goal has been met. No improvement goal is included in this statement; rather, it is a restatement of targeted performance. The pitfalls of this statement include the risk of micromanaging the activities that occur at the patient encounter rather than improving the underlying work process (i.e., the focus is on the operational activities, not on an improvement process). In addition, the manager again risks "getting what he asks for" (i.e., an exclusive focus on immunizations).

Multiple Goals. *Track patient compliance with well-child exams. Notify and schedule patients who have missed well-child exams. Give age-appropriate immunizations during well-child exams.*

At first glance, this goal statement also might appear to be effective; however, it reflects a solution, not a goal. Because these statements are specific interventions to be carried out, this type of goal would be appropriate to describe new work expectations for care providers once the improved process has been designed. Differentiate between implementation goals (i.e., behavior expectations or guidelines for implementing a predetermined intervention) and goals for an improvement effort (i.e., to identify/design interventions that will lead to improved performance) to ensure that the goal statement is consistent with the purpose/intent.

Implicit Goal/General Goal. *Improve immunization rates.*

The statement "improve immunization rates" may be considered an implicit goal or a general goal. Often, goals are stated in general terms, such as "improve the quality of care." Instead, try posing the question, "If I knew nothing about the problem and you gave me this goal, could you be sure that you would get the results that you desired when I was 'done'?" If the answer to this question is no, implicit goals that need to be made explicit are likely hidden in the statement. General goals may be appropriate for setting overall direction for a team/department/organization; however, more specific direction will help ensure success of an improvement effort.

Simple Goal. *Give age-appropriate immunizations at each well-child appointment.*

Although this may appear to be an effective goal, the major pitfall of this goal statement is that it limits the nature of the improvements. For example, by stating the goal in this way, interventions will most likely be limited to the well-child appointment. Opportunities to combine sick-child visits with preventive care may be not be considered, and children who miss well-child appointments may be overlooked.

Unclear Goal. *Work with the office staff to improve pediatric care.*

With an unclear goal such as this one, the goal may be met but the desired results not achieved. Because the goal is vague, efforts may be taken to meet this goal that improve pediatric care (e.g., care of patients with asthma) but not address the problem of immunization rates.

Negative Goal. *Reduce the number of patients with incomplete immunizations.*

Negative language leads one to focus on problems rather than solutions, which could dampen the motivation of those participating in the improvement effort.

SMART Goals and Complex Systems

Revisiting SMART (specific, measurable, achievable, relevant, and time-framed) goals within the context of quality management in complex systems yields the following lessons.

Specific

Goals should be specific enough to give direction; however, if improvement goals are too specific, they may limit the opportunity for improvement. When working in complex systems, a general goal statement used as a partial or intermediate goal is appropriate if there is inadequate information about the problem.

Measurable

If improvement goals are limited to only those areas that one can measure, improvement efforts are confined by one's current abilities. As quality and improvement skills mature, so should our ability to define and measure quality. Sometimes in improvement efforts, developing the measure is part of the effort.

Achievable

If improvement goals are limited to the perception of what is achievable, the potential for innovative or breakthrough solutions is also limited. While including numeric targets at the strategic level is common practice and perhaps necessary, such inclusion risks placing a ceiling on the improvement effort. For example, staff may stop improvement efforts at the target of 3 percent rather than seeking the innovative solution that could result in 20 percent improvement. In complex systems, monitoring the ongoing performance and variability over time is more important than focusing on a static target.

Relevant

What is perceived as relevant from one perspective may not be relevant when viewed from another perspective. Perspective and context are required to determine relevance and are a prerequisite to setting appropriate goals.

Time-Framed

Improvement should be continuous. Expectations about implementing interventions may be time-framed; however, performance of the system is dependent on the underlying structures of the system. If a goal does not address systemic causes of the problem, a time frame can set up the effort to fail rather than promote its success.

Corollaries to Purpose and Goals

Purpose and goals go hand in hand when viewing quality management from a systems perspective. The corollaries represented in the following questions can help managers understand the complete picture.

- What is the *purpose?* (Why does "it" exist?)
- What are the desired *results?* (How is the successful accomplishment of the purpose defined?)
- What *activities* are used to accomplish the purpose? (What are the processes and interventions to achieve the purpose?)
- How is the accomplishment of the purpose *measured?* (How does one determine how well the purpose is being accomplished?)
- What are the improvement *goals?* (How does one improve how well the purpose is being accomplished?)

Revisiting the Chapter 5 example on prenatal services illustrates these corollaries.

- The *purpose* of the clinic's prenatal services is to assess, monitor, and manage the physiological and psychosocial needs of families during the childbearing process.
- The desired *results* are healthy clinical outcomes, satisfied patients, and cost-effective services.
- The clinic will *measure* its success in achieving the desired results with the following data: maternal and infant complication rates, early diagnosis rates, patient satisfaction, payer satisfaction, and so on.
- The *service mix, processes, and interventions* used to accomplish the purpose are strategically determined, designed, and improved.
- The *goal* for improvement efforts may be to validate the purposes of the key stakeholders identified earlier; refine the clinic's purpose for prenatal care services based on any new information obtained; evaluate current practices to determine the extent to which the clinic is accomplishing its purpose; define a service mix that is consistent with the purpose; prioritize those services needing improvement; and design, redesign, and implement improved processes that meet all stakeholder requirements and accomplish the new definition of purpose. (This is a multiple, positive, clear goal incorporating partial or intermediate goals.)

Even those experienced in quality improvement may set goals based on ingrained habits and find setting goals from a systems perspective counterintuitive. For example, a quality improvement workshop advertises this way: "Improving Your HCAHPS Score Through Patient-Centered Care" (IHI 2009). An understanding of systems thinking would reframe this statement to: "Improve your organization's ability to deliver patient-centered care as *measured* by your HCAHPS scores."

Summary

Effective goals precede effective performance. Familiar mental models concerning goals are represented in SMART goals and how goals and objectives are defined within the context of program planning. This chapter has explored mental models from the perspective of improvement within complex systems and techniques managers may use to improve their own goal-setting skills. Although no single correct or incorrect approach to setting a goal exists, managers should be aware of the advantages and pitfalls of each approach and the ways the goals are communicated. To enhance their effectiveness in setting improvement goals within the context of complex systems, managers should (Kelly 2009a):

- differentiate between improvement goals and operational expectations;
- clarify the difference between solutions, goals, action plans, and improvement efforts;
- address underlying work processes that lead to results;
- leverage like processes;
- remember that setting a goal is different from measuring how effectively one is meeting the goal; and
- use intermediate goals and revise as new information is gathered.

Exercise

Objective: To practice linking goal statements with results.

Scenario:
Many researchers use the CMS database. One study of the first set of Hospital Quality Alliance–reported quality indicators found the following results:

> Analysis of data from the Hospital Quality Alliance national reporting system shows that performance varies among hospitals and across indicators. . . . [P]erformance scores for acute myocardial infarction closely predicted performance scores for congestive health failure but not for pneumonia. . . . [O]ur findings indicate that quality measures had only moderate predictive ability across the three conditions. Although a high quality of care for acute myocardial infarction predicted a high quality of care for congestive heart failure, the former was only marginally better than chance for identifying a high quality of care for pneumonia. These data do not provide support for the notion that 'good' hospitals are easy to identify or consistent in their performance across conditions. (Jha et al. 2005, 265, 272)

For the purposes of this exercise, assume the unit of analysis in the preceding paragraph is one hospital rather than a collective group of Hospital Quality Alliance participants. The results suggest that the hospital approached the improvements in a fragmented, disease-specific manner.

Instructions:

Consider how organizational goals may have contributed to some improvement in congestive heart failure and acute MI care while improvements in pneumonia lagged.

Write one goal statement that the hospital could have established that would have led to the results described. Critique the goal statement and document your critique on a worksheet such as the one below. Remember, you are critiquing the goal statement, not the merit of the intervention represented by the goal statement.

Write a second goal statement that the hospital could have established that would have led to the different results. Critique the goal statement and document your critique on a worksheet such as the one below. Remember, you are critiquing the goal statement, not the merit of the intervention represented by the goal statement.

Goals Worksheet

Goal Statement	Type of Goal	Pros	Cons

Companion Readings

Dorner, D. 1996. *The Logic of Failure: Recognizing and Avoiding Error in Complex Situations*, 49–70. Reading, MA: Perseus Books.

Klein, G., and K. E. Weick. 2000. "Decisions: Making the Right Ones, Learning from the Wrong Ones." *Across the Board* 37 (6): 16–22. [Online article.] www.conference-board.org/articles/atb_article.cfm?id=96.

Web Resources

New England Complex System Institute: About Complex Systems
   www.necsi.edu/guide/
High-Reliability.org: Managing the Unexpected
   http://high-reliability.org/

UNDERSTANDING CUSTOMER AND STAKEHOLDER REQUIREMENTS

Learning Objectives

After completing this chapter you should be able to:

- define patient expectations according to research conducted by the Picker Institute;
- begin to translate patient/client/customer requirements into service features and organizational processes;
- explain the goals and uses of the Consumer Assessment of Healthcare Providers and Systems programs;
- demonstrate the value of patient perceptions data to organizational change from a systems perspective; and
- link accreditation and consumer requirements to managerial responsibilities within a health services organization.

The new mother explained, "The morning after I had my baby, I remember holding my toothbrush in my hand for over an hour. Every few minutes, someone else knocked on the door and without waiting for me to answer, entered my room: the doctor, the nurse, another nurse, the birth certificate recorder, the person collecting the meal menu, someone inviting me to attend a baby bath class. They all wanted something. I just wanted to brush my teeth!"

Demonstrating interpersonal behaviors such as courtesy is essential to a satisfying patient or client experience. Organizational factors (e.g., coordination of services) are also associated with a satisfying experience. Coordination is often thought of within the context of the medical treatment plan between physicians; nursing care across hospital shifts; scheduling of appointments for diagnostic exams; and interventions between health services disciplines. These areas of coordination are all important from the technical perspective of quality. Missing in the example is coordination from the patient's experience perspective. While each individual encounter with the new mother in our example may have been positive, the collective experience from the patient's perspective was not.

Understanding patients, clients, customers, and stakeholders is essential if managers are to design organizational processes that meet their requirements.

Patient Requirements

Asking and observing are the most informal ways to identify patient needs and expectations. Simple questions such as "What brought you to the office today?" or "Can you describe your pain?" can help frontline care providers understand the patient's immediate needs and take action to meet them.

While those with the direct customer interface must be concerned with individual patient requirements, managers must also be concerned with these individuals within the context of customer groups served by the organization. Patient-focused approaches require an understanding not only of who the customers are but also of what these customers require; how the requirements differ between customer groups; how these requirements change over time; and how these requirements guide organizational strategy, decisions, and activities (National Institute of Standards and Technology 2011).

Patients as customer groups may be differentiated by disease category (e.g., cancer, cardiovascular, obstetrics), age, the nature of the illness (e.g., chronic, acute), the site of care (e.g., inpatient, outpatient, long-term care), ethnicity, or language. The advent of evening outpatient clinic hours illustrates how organizational decisions on hours of operation have changed to keep pace with changing patient work schedules. Adopting culturally competent approaches to patient care, incorporating translation services, and providing patient education materials in multiple languages are examples of how organizations have adapted their internal operations to meet the needs of ethnically diverse communities.

Scanning the published literature for information on customer expectations can help a manager avoid reinventing the wheel. For example, the Picker Institute was established in 1987 to promote patient-focused care and to provide information to health services organizations about patient-focused approaches. On the basis of information obtained from focus groups, literature, and health professionals, the Picker Institute (2010) has identified and defined specific patient requirements, also called dimensions or principles of patient-focused care:

- Respect for patients' values, preferences, and expressed needs
- Coordination and integration of care
- Information, communication, and education
- Physical comfort
- Emotional support and alleviation of fear and anxiety
- Involvement of family and friends

- Continuity and transition
- Access to care

These dimensions of care described by the Picker Institute provide an excellent starting point for any health services manager to begin a customer-focused improvement effort. Depending on the organization's needs and resources, a deeper understanding of patient requirements may be obtained through focus groups and other qualitative research methods.

Once patient expectations and requirements are known, they must be translated into product or service features to ensure that they are being met on a consistent basis for all customers who interact with that product or service. As consumers, many readers are already acquainted with this concept. Smart phones are examples of improvements to telecommunications, incorporating features and applications to meet customer expectations in the digital information age. Experienced health services organizations are continually improving their abilities to translate patient expectations into service and product features.

Translating the dimensions of care into service features is illustrated by an oral surgeon who is a favorite among teenage patients and families for removing wisdom teeth in the office setting (Exhibit 7.1). The entire patient experience from beginning to end demonstrates his understanding of patient requirements and his commitment to design of office space, surgical procedures, and service experience to meet those requirements.

While much progress has been made, not all providers have embraced the philosophy of customer focus. Chapter 1 described Donabedian's dual nature of medical quality: the combination of technical and interpersonal components for a comprehensive view of quality care. Managers must remember that many health services professionals have been educated in a philosophy that defines quality according to the professional's expertise and expectations rather than according to the patient's expectations or requirements. The term **technical quality** refers to clinical expertise and technical aspects of healthcare (e.g., selecting the appropriate intervention for a patient's symptoms or carrying out a clinical procedure properly). Most patients assume that providers possess and deliver technical quality. The term **service quality** refers to the "myriad characteristics that shape the experience of care for patients" (Kenagy, Berwick, and Shore 1999, 661), including interpersonal components of care (e.g., empathy and communication) and how well a patient's requirements and expectations are being met (e.g., access, timeliness).

Managers should determine the extent to which they themselves, as well as providers and other employees, understand and accept the dual nature of quality. Managers, as departmental or organizational leaders, are responsible for establishing a customer-focused environment and direction for their employees. This comment from a skilled technical nurse—"I wish

Technical quality
clinical expertise and technical aspects of healthcare

Service quality
the "myriad characteristics that shape the experience of care for patients" (Kenagy, Berwick, and Shore 1999, 661) including interpersonal components of care (e.g., empathy and communication) and how well a patient's requirements and expectations are being met

EXHIBIT 7.1

Translating Dimensions of Care into Service Features

Patient Requirement	Service Feature
Access to care	The oral surgeon established referral relationships with orthodontists in the area according to location and patient's specific insurance coverage.
Coordination and integration of care	The oral surgeon and orthodontists have formalized communication practices to coordinate with each other and with the family about the referral.
Respect for patients' values, preferences, and expressed needs	The oral surgeon offers flexibility in scheduling the appointment date and time according to students' school and activity schedules.
Information and education	The day before the procedure, the oral surgeon's staff call the parents to confirm the appointment, give pre-operative instructions, and answer questions. Immediately after the procedure, the staff give the parents postoperative instructions verbally and also in writing.
Physical comfort	The office contains comfortable furniture; the patient is carefully positioned during surgery; pain management is provided during the procedure and after discharge.
Involvement of family and friends	The parents are invited to accompany the patient to the procedure room and to stay until the patient's sedation takes effect. The parents are provided with estimated length of procedure time and notified when the procedure is completed.
Emotional support and alleviation of fear and anxiety	The waiting room is decorated in a soothing color scheme and includes a water feature and fish tank. The staff patiently answer all of the parents' questions regarding surgeon qualifications, anesthesia safety, and procedures in case of an emergency. The surgeon's communication style demonstrates his knowledge of and rapport with teenage clients.
Transition and continuity	A follow-up appointment is made before the patient leaves the office. A follow-up phone call is made by the surgeon the evening of the surgery.

the family would get out of the way so I could do my job"—suggests a work environment in which content quality is valued and rewarded above service quality. An understanding of systemic structure (Chapter 3) helps managers see that policies and procedures, job descriptions, personnel performance expectations and evaluations, reward systems, and staff development may create and sustain a customer-focused environment. By purposefully and strategically incorporating both aspects of quality care into the design of these management tools, managers may enhance their ability to implement a focus on both content quality and service quality.

Measuring Patient Perceptions of Care

Numerous vendor-designed and home-grown instruments have been used in the past in an attempt to capture patient satisfaction data. Unfortunately, the methods had little comparability between sites of care. The Centers for Medicare & Medicaid Services (CMS) and the Agency for Health-care Research and Quality (AHRQ) jointly developed and tested the first national instrument and methodology to directly survey patients' perception of care. The Consumer Assessment of Health Providers and Systems (CAHPS) was first implemented in the hospital setting on a voluntary basis in 2006 and then required as part of CMS's *Reporting Hospital Quality Data for Annual Payment Update* program (RHQDAPU) in 2008 (see Chapter 8). As a result, hospitals rapidly adopted the Hospital CAHPS (HCAHPS), and in 2009, 98 percent of US acute care hospitals participated in the program (CMS 2010b, Giordano et al. 2010). Exhibit 7.2 presents a summary of the HCAHPS program. Exhibit 7.3 presents the care-related questions that accompany several demographic questions. The influence of the dimensions of care defined by the Picker Institute is notable throughout these questions.

The CAHPS instrument is now available for other settings of care, including a variety of ambulatory care settings, hemodialysis centers, and nursing homes (AHRQ 2010a). Results of the HCAHPS surveys are reported on the CMS Hospital Compare website (CMS 2010b) and are updated quarterly. The analyzed data are available to the public and researchers.

Implications for Managers

Consider how a manager might respond to HCAHPS results within the context of the iceberg metaphor of organizations as systems (Chapter 3). An event-level response would be to design improvements for individual questions for which results did not meet expectations. For example, if the question, *Before giving you any new medicine, how often did hospital staff describe possible side effects in a way you could understand?* showed a low score, the manager might implement a new policy. He could buy education pamphlets about the side effects of every medication on the hospital's formulary, and require staff to give patients a medication pamphlet when a drug is given for the first time. Responding at the events level (i.e., to individual indicator results) leads to a flurry of activity and an overwhelmed staff faced with a barrage of new policies and does little to increase the organization's ability to adapt its operations as new requirements are published.

A patterns-level response within the context of the iceberg metaphor would explore a combination of similar questions. For example, several

HCAHPS questions involve explaining or providing new information to patients:

- During this hospital stay, how often did nurses explain things in a way you could understand?
- During this hospital stay, how often did doctors explain things in a way you could understand?
- Before giving you any new medicine, how often did hospital staff tell you what the medicine was for?
- Before giving you any new medicine, how often did hospital staff describe possible side effects in a way you could understand?
- During this hospital stay, did doctors, nurses, or other hospital staff talk with you about whether you would have the help you needed when you left the hospital?
- During this hospital stay, did you get information in writing about what symptoms or health problems to look out for after you left the hospital?

Analyzing these questions collectively gives the manager more information and prompts new questions on which to guide improvement decisions. Why does one question score much lower than others? Why do the discharge questions score higher than the questions about explaining things throughout the hospital stay? Do we use written or verbal approaches? Is there a standardized system for patient education? Understanding the patterns allows the manager to leverage improvements to address multiple questions with similar causes; in this case, ensuring a patient education system, using a variety of methods based on patient needs and learning styles, is embedded in the patient's plan of care.

While managers look for patterns within the organization, researchers use the HCAHPS data to identify patterns between organizations. Studies of the publicly reported clinical quality measures with the HCAHPS data are beginning to show associations between technical quality of care and patient perceptions of care (Isaac et al. 2010; Taylor et al. 2008; Jha et al. 2008).

Analyzing the HCAHPS data from below the waterline encourages the manager to search for system structures. For example, when viewed collectively and over time, the HCAHPS data provide managers with valuable information about the patient's experience with the organization as a measure of the organization's culture (Framptom and Wahl 2010). Culture has also been related to patient safety (Sammer et al. 2010; Reiman, Pietikäinen, and Oedewald 2010). The link between patient perceptions and technical quality becomes clearer when one realizes the role of culture as a systemic structure influencing organizational results and the shared characteristics of a patient-focused culture and a safety culture.

As described in Chapter 1, understanding the organization (in this case organizational culture) guides managers in improving organizations.

The CAHPS Hospital Survey, also known as Hospital CAHPS or HCAHPS, is a standardized survey instrument and data collection methodology for measuring patients' perspectives of hospital care.

While many hospitals collect information on patient satisfaction, no national standard for collecting or publicly reporting this information exists that would enable valid comparisons to be made across all hospitals. To make "apples to apples" comparisons to support consumer choice, a standard measurement approach must be introduced. HCAHPS is a core set of questions that can be combined with customized, hospital-specific items to produce information that complements the data hospitals currently collect to support internal customer service and quality-related activities.

Three broad goals have shaped the HCAHPS survey. First, the survey is designed to produce comparable data on patients' perspectives of care that allows objective and meaningful comparisons among hospitals on topics that are important to consumers. Second, public reporting of the survey results is designed to create incentives for hospitals to improve quality of care. Third, public reporting will serve to enhance public accountability in healthcare by increasing the transparency of the quality of hospital care provided in return for the public investment. With these goals in mind, the HCAHPS project has taken substantial steps to ensure that the survey is credible, useful, and practical. This methodology and the information it generates will be made available to the public.

The Centers for Medicare & Medicaid Services (CMS) partnered with the Agency for Healthcare Research and Quality (AHRQ), another agency in the Department of Health and Human Services, to develop HCAHPS. AHRQ carried out a rigorous scientific process to develop and test the HCAHPS instrument. This process entailed multiple steps, including a public call for measures; literature review; cognitive interviews; consumer focus groups; stakeholder input; a three-state pilot test; consumer testing; small-scale field tests; and responding to public comments generated by several *Federal Register* notices.

Voluntary collection of HCAHPS data for public reporting began in October 2006. The first public reporting of HCAHPS results, which encompassed eligible discharges from October 2006 through June 2007, occurred in March 2008.

Source: CMS (2010b).

EXHIBIT 7.2
HCAHPS:
Hospital
Consumer
Assessment
of Healthcare
Providers
and Systems
Background

Improvement interventions that target culture (systemic structure) may then be selected (Charmel 2010; Cliff 2010; Shortell and Singer 2008; Skyve 2009; Caldwell 2008; Jiang et al. 2008; Shorr 2007). The key lesson for health services organizations is that leadership is the leverage to truly transform patient perceptions *and* clinical quality. The cascading influence of board and leadership decisions may then infiltrate all other levels of management throughout the organization to bring about cultural change. As described in Chapter 3, sustainable change is only possible by changing the fundamental system behavior.

EXHIBIT 7.3
HCAHPS:
Hospital
Consumer
Assessment
of Healthcare
Providers and
Systems Survey
Questions

- During this hospital stay, how often did nurses treat you with *courtesy and respect*?
- During this hospital stay, how often did nurses *listen carefully to you*?
- During this hospital stay, how often did nurses *explain things* in a way you could understand?
- During this hospital stay, after you pressed the call button, how often did you get help as soon as you wanted it?
- During this hospital stay, how often did doctors treat you with *courtesy and respect*?
- During this hospital stay, how often did doctors *listen carefully to you*?
- During this hospital stay, how often did doctors *explain things* in a way you could understand?
- During this hospital stay, how often were your room and bathroom kept clean?
- During this hospital stay, how often was the area around your room quiet at night?
- How often did you get help in getting to the bathroom or in using a bedpan as soon as you wanted?
- During this hospital stay, how often was your pain well controlled?
- During this hospital stay, how often did the hospital staff do everything they could to help you with your pain?
- Before giving you any new medicine, how often did hospital staff tell you what the medicine was for?
- Before giving you any new medicine, how often did hospital staff describe possible side effects in a way you could understand?
- During this hospital stay, did doctors, nurses, or other hospital staff talk with you about whether you would have the help you needed when you left the hospital?
- During this hospital stay, did you get information in writing about what symptoms or health problems to look out for after you left the hospital?
- Using any number from 0 to 10, where 0 is the worst hospital possible and 10 is the best hospital possible, what number would you use to rate this hospital during your stay?
- Would you recommend this hospital to your friends and family?

Source: HCAHPS (2010).

Managers are essential to align, implement, and institutionalize organizational processes and working conditions that reflect and foster desired organizational characteristics and personal behaviors. From this perspective, the management function of "staffing" may be viewed as an important cultural tool:

> Eleven years ago, I [Diane Kelly] was quoted in the *Wall Street Journal* as saying, "We hold people's lives in our hands at a very vulnerable time . . . healthcare is about a personal encounter" (Petzinger 1998, B1). . . . Since that time, I have come to better appreciate the crucial role of leadership at all decision-making levels of health ser-

vices organizations in establishing organizational direction, *allocating resources*, and designing metrics that support the personal encounter. A commitment to purposefully paying attention to the interaction, to the person, in the moment, drives behavior within the personal and organizational context in which care is provided. Some refer to this as "mindfulness," which may be compared to ideas of situational awareness, group climate, and interpersonal relationship described in the human factors [and safety] literature. By increasing our personal skills in paying attention, we can concurrently advance both patient-centeredness and patient safety. (Kelly 2009c)

Beyond Service Quality: Meeting Stakeholder Requirements

As discussed in Chapter 1, a customer is an actual or potential user of services; the contemporary view of quality management expands the concept of "customer" to include stakeholders and markets in which the organization operates. The stakeholders of health services organizations are numerous and diverse. The manager is responsible for identifying the stakeholders of a specific organization, program, or service as well as their requirements.

Accreditation bodies, federal and state governments, and private organizations such as the National Quality Forum are examples of stakeholders whose requirements for health services organizations are changing and evolving. The topics of "transparency" and quality reporting are discussed in more detail in Chapter 8. Two stakeholder initiatives are discussed here: The Joint Commission's National Patient Safety Goals and practices recommended by the Leapfrog Group.

The Joint Commission

The Joint Commission is a private accreditation body for numerous types of healthcare delivery organizations (see Chapter 8). In 1996, The Joint Commission implemented its sentinel event policy for hospitals (The Joint Commission 2009a). A **sentinel event** is defined by The Joint Commission (2010f) as

> an unexpected occurrence involving death or serious physical or psychological injury, or the risk thereof. Serious injury specifically includes loss of limb or function. The phrase, "or the risk thereof" includes any process variation for which a recurrence would carry a significant chance of a serious adverse outcome. Such events are called "sentinel" because they signal the need for immediate investigation and response.

When a sentinel event occurs, the policy requires Joint Commission–accredited hospitals to conduct a **root cause analysis** (RCA). Results of the RCAs are collected and analyzed in the Sentinel Event Data Base. Using published clinical research results combined with the Sentinel Event Data Base analysis results, The Joint Commission developed and implemented the

The Joint Commission
a private accreditation body for numerous types of services organizations

Sentinel event
"an unexpected occurrence involving death or serious physical or psychological injury, or the risk thereof. Serious injury specifically includes loss of limb or function" (The Joint Commission 2010f)

Root cause analysis (RCA)
"a process for identifying basic or causal factor(s) underlying variation in performance, including the occurrence or possible occurrence of a sentinel event" (Croteau 2010)

National Patient Safety Goals (NPSGs) program. The first set of NPSGs went into effect in 2003 and has evolved to include nine settings of care: ambulatory healthcare, behavioral health care, critical access hospitals, home care, hospitals, laboratories, long-term care, Medicare/Medicaid long-term care, and office-based care (The Joint Commission 2010a). The Joint Commission applies a continuous improvement approach to the NPSGs demonstrated through its annual review process. Annual changes are designed to "focus the NPSGs on those topics that are of highest priority to patient safety and quality care" (The Joint Commission 2009a). As the required safe practice becomes widely adopted and it "is no longer necessary to 'spotlight' the issue in the NPSGs," the practice moves from the status of an NPSG to a standard.

The NPSGs compel system change through below-the-waterline questions about core managerial responsibilities and decisions. For example, since their first implementation, NPSGs have had implications for how managers make decisions about capital equipment (e.g., infusion pumps), preventive maintenance (e.g., maintenance of patient monitors), procurement (e.g., pharmaceuticals), and training (e.g., Centers for Disease Control and Prevention hand-washing guidelines). The NPSGs have implications for how managers prioritize improvements (e.g., fall-reduction program), establish communication systems between departments (e.g., between laboratory staff and care providers), establish communication between sites of care (e.g., medication reconciliation), and evaluate documentation tools (e.g., "do not use" abbreviations).

The Leapfrog Group

The role of payers as stakeholders in the quality agenda has also evolved in recent years. In addition to insurance companies and government programs such as Medicare, employers who provide health insurance as an employee benefit must also be considered "payers." The Leapfrog Group is one of the most influential of this type of stakeholder. The Leapfrog Group (2010, 1) is a

> growing consortium of major companies and other large private and public healthcare purchasers that provide health benefits to more than 37 million Americans in all 50 states. Leapfrog members and their employees spend tens of billions of dollars on health care annually. Leapfrog members agree to base their purchase of health care on principles that encourage quality improvement among providers and consumer involvement in health care decision making.

Leapfrog members have endorsed specific safe practices as negotiating points between employers and health plans. These are

> Computerized Physician Order Entry (CPOE): With CPOE systems, hospital staff enter medication orders via computers linked to software designed to prevent prescribing errors. CPOE has been shown to reduce serious prescribing errors by more than 50%.

Evidence-Based Hospital Referral (EHR): Consumers and health care purchasers should choose hospitals with the best track records. By referring patients needing certain complex medical procedures to hospitals offering the best survival odds based on scientifically valid criteria—such as the number of times a hospital performs a procedure each year or other process or outcomes data—studies indicate that a patient's risk of dying could be significantly reduced.

ICU Physician Staffing (IPS): Staffing ICUs with intensivists—doctors who have special training in critical care medicine—has been shown to reduce the risk of patients dying in the ICU by 40%.

Leapfrog Safe Practices Score: The National Quality Forum–endorsed Safe Practices cover a range of practices that, if utilized, would reduce the risk of harm in certain processes, systems or environments of care. Included in the 34 practices are the three leaps above. This fourth leap assesses a hospital's progress on 17 of the remaining 31 NQF safe practices. (Leapfrog Group 2010, 2)

As with the NPSGs, meeting the Leapfrog Group's requirements forces managers to evaluate and change core responsibilities and decisions as well as the assumptions on which organizational decisions are based. The Leapfrog Group's requirements are important for managers to consider in the areas of capital planning and investment (e.g., computerized physician order entry), human resources management and physician relations (e.g., intensivists), service mix and revenue sources (e.g., evidence-based hospital referrals), and operational transparency (e.g., Leapfrog Safe Practices Score).

Summary

The traditional concept of "the customer" has expanded to include the contemporary view of stakeholders and markets in which an organization operates. Patient and customer requirements from health services organizations have been studied and documented, and are now being measured and reported on a national scale in the United States. Stakeholders of health services organizations are numerous and diverse with continually changing and evolving requirements. Managers must keep abreast of changes in existing and emerging requirements and their influence on their organizational responsibilities, and the accompanying value in promoting below-the-waterline improvements.

Exercise

Objective:
Practice identifying management behaviors that demonstrate a focus on customers.

Instructions:
- Read the case study.
- Describe several ways that management demonstrated a focus on customers throughout this case study.

Case Study:

The following account of an improvement effort in an ambulatory surgery unit is told by the former *Wall Street Journal* columnist Thomas Petzinger, Jr.

While many companies are getting better at customer service, one industry has gotten a lot worse lately. That industry is medicine. The onslaught of managed care has commoditized what was once the most delicate relationship in all of commerce, that of doctor and patient. Accounting for the payment of services has overwhelmed the rendering of the services themselves. Yet a few islands of people have thrown off their Newtonian blinders and recognized that putting the customer first can redound to the benefit of the provider as well. With so many competing claims on every dollar, every process, and every hour of time and attention, the interests of the customer—the patient—serve as a common ground for making the entire system more efficient.

One hospital is such a place: a 520-bed teaching hospital and so-called trauma-one center with a stellar clinical reputation. Within the hospital, an outpatient surgery clinic was opened long ago, in which an ever-larger percentage of procedures were being conducted. And although the surgical staff was acclaimed, management recognized that the overall patient experience left something to be desired.

The main problem was delay. The surgery line was jam-packed as early as 5:30 every morning. Some patients spent the entire day lurching from check-in to pre-op to anesthesia to surgery to recovery to post-op, with too much of the time spent simply waiting. As much as some people may wish to convalesce at length as admitted hospital patients, no one wants to turn a four-hour outpatient experience into a nine-hour ordeal. If the hospital wanted to maintain (much less extend) its position in the marketplace, it had to figure out how to get patients through faster without degrading clinical results.

The job of facilitating the planning process went to an internal quality consultant who had worked for 15 years as a registered nurse, mostly in neonatal intensive care, before earning her MBA and fulfilling this new organizational role. In her years in intensive care, she was often perplexed by the priorities that families exhibited in the most dire medical situations. "I'm working like crazy to save a baby, but the parents get upset because the grandparents didn't get to see the baby!" she recalls. In time she could see that medicine was only part of healthcare. "Healthcare providers hold people's lives in their hands at a very vulnerable time," she says. "Healthcare is about a personal encounter." Most of the people on the business side of healthcare have little intellectual grasp and less emotional grasp of this concept. Indeed, after moving to the business side herself, she became convinced that some of the most intractable problems of the industry could be solved only by people who, like her, combined far-flung disciplines. "Innovation will come from people who have crossed the boundaries from other disciplines," she says—from business to medicine, from medicine to law, and so on.

The facilitator insisted on involving the maximum number of nurses—people who knew the whole patient as well as the individual surgeries they variously received. The new administrator over the area requested that the members of the improvement committee visit as many other hospitals as possible within their large hospital system to explore which outpatient surgical practices could be employed at their own site. And throughout the study process, the administrator continually harped on the "vision statement" of the initiative, which put as its first priority "to provide a patient/family focused quality culture."

This new administrator in the surgery service, a nurse herself, was a powerful force in leading the improvement effort. Under the previous leadership, the policy for change was simply "give the surgeons whatever they want," as she put it. The administrator acknowledged that the surgeon must call the shots on procedures—but not necessarily on process. In that respect she, too, insisted on using the patient as the point of departure. "If you're guided by only one phrase—what is best for the patient—you will always come up with the right answer," the administrator insists. (Hearing the administrator and facilitator say this over and over began to remind me of the best editors I have worked for. When in doubt, they would often say, do only what's right for the reader. Everything else will fall into place.)

Studying the surgery line from the patients' point of view was disturbingly illuminating. Surgeons showing up late for the first round of surgeries at 7:30 am threw off the schedule for the entire day. The various hospital departments—admitting, financing, lab, surgery—all conducted their own separate interaction with the patient on each of their individual schedules. A poor physical layout, including a long corridor separating the operating rooms from pre-op, compounded the inefficiencies. Once a patient was called to surgery, he spent 40 minutes waiting for an orderly to arrive with a wheelchair or gurney. And, because this was an outpatient surgery center located inside a hospital, the anesthesiologists were accustomed to administering heavy sedation, often slowing the patient's recovery from otherwise minor surgery and further clogging the entire line. The operation was a success, but the patient was pissed.

In talking to patients, the researchers discovered a subtext in the complaints about delays: resentment over the loss of personal control. Patients spent the day in God-awful gauze gowns, stripped of their underwear, their backsides exposed to the world. Partly this reflected a medical culture that considered the procedure, not the patient, as the customer. As the administrator put it to me, "If you're naked on a stretcher on your back, you're pretty subservient." Family members, meanwhile, had to roam the hospital in search of change so they could coax a cup of coffee from a vending machine. She marveled at the arrogance of it. "You're spending $3,000 on a loved one, but you'd better bring correct change."

Fortunately, this administrator had the political standing to push through big changes, and although the staff surgeons effectively had veto power, most were too busy to get deeply involved in the improvement process. Because few patients enjoy getting stuck with needles, the nurses created a process for capturing the blood from the insertion of each patient's intravenous needle and sending it to the lab for whatever tests were necessary. This cut down not only on discomfort, but on time, money, and scheduling complexity. The unremitting bureaucratic questions and paperwork were all replaced with a single registration packet that patients picked up in their doctors' offices and completed days before ever setting foot in the hospital; last-minute administrative details were attended to in a single phone call the day before surgery. The nurses set up a check-in system for the coats and valuables of patients and family members, which eliminated the need for every family to encamp with their belongings in a pre-op room for the entire day. A family-friendly waiting area was created, stocked with free snacks and drinks. There would be no more desperate searches for correct change.

That was only the beginning. Patients had always resented having to purchase their post-op medications from the hospital pharmacy; simply freeing them to use their neighborhood drugstore got them out of the surgery line sooner, further relieving the congestion. Also in the interest of saving time, the nurses made a heretical proposal to allow healthy outpatients to walk into surgery under their own power, accompanied by their family members, rather than waiting 40 minutes for a wheelchair or gurney. That idea got the attention of the surgeons, who after years of paying ghastly malpractice premiums vowed that the administrator, not they, would suffer the personal liability on that one. The risk-management department went "eek" at the idea. Yet as the improvement committee pointed out, the hospital permitted outpatients to traverse any other distance in the building by foot. Why should the march into surgery be any different?

In a similar vein, the nurses suggested allowing patients to wear underwear beneath their hospital gowns. The administrators could scarcely believe their ears: "Show me one place in the literature where patients wear underwear to surgery!" one top administrator demanded. (The nurses noted that restricting change to what had been attempted elsewhere would automatically eliminate the possibility of any breakthrough in performance.) And why stop at underwear, the nurses asked. The hospital was conducting more and more outpatient cataract operations; why not let these patients wear their clothes into surgery? "Contamination!" the purists cried. But clothing is no dirtier than the skin beneath it, the nurses answered. This change eliminated a major post-op bottleneck caused by elderly patients who could not dress themselves or tie their shoes with their heads clouded by anesthesia and their depth perception altered by the removal of their cataracts.

As the changes took effect, the nurses observed another unintended effect. Patients were actually reducing their recovery times! People were no longer looking at ceiling tiles on their way into surgery like characters in an episode of *Dr. Kildare*. They went into surgery feeling better and came out of it feeling better. In case after case they were ready to leave the joint faster, which in turn freed up more space for other patients. Because they had studied practices at a number of stand-alone clinics, the nurses even suggested to the physicians that the outpatients would be better off with less anesthesia, hastening their recoveries, speeding their exit, and freeing up still more capacity.

Within a year, the volume at the outpatient surgery unit had surged 50 percent with no increase in square footage and no increase in staff. Customer-service surveys were positive and costs were under control. And it dawned on the facilitator that the nurses' intuitive conviction that the patient should come first benefited the surgery line itself at every single step. Everyone and everything connected to the process—surgeon, staff, insurers, time, cost, and quality—seemed to come out ahead when the patients' interests came first.

What was really happening, of course, was that the change teams simply put common sense first. In a complex process of many players, the interest of the patient was the one unifying characteristic—the best baseline for calibration—because the patient was the only person touched by every step.

Reprinted with slight changes with the permission of Simon & Schuster Adult Publishing Group from *The New Pioneers: The Men and Women Who Are Transforming the Workplace and Marketplace* by Thomas Petzinger, Jr. Copyright © 1999 by Thomas Petzinger, Jr.

Companion Readings

Cliff, B. 2010. "The Leadership Journey of Patient-Centered Care." *Frontiers of Health Services Management* 26 (4): 35–39.

Isaac, T., A. M. Zaslavsky, P. D. Cleary, and B. E. Landon. 2010. "The Relationship Between Patients' Perception of Care and Measures of Hospital Quality and Safety." *Health Services Research* 45 (4): 1024–40.

Weick, K. E., and T. Putnam. 2006. "Organizing for Mindfulness: Eastern Wisdom and Western Knowledge." *Journal of Management Inquiry* 15 (3): 275–87.

Web Resources

The Joint Commission: www.jointcommission.org

The Joint Commission International Center for Patient Safety:
www.jcipatientsafety.org

The Joint Commission National Patient Safety Goals:
www.jointcommission.org/PatientSafety/NationalPatientSafetyGoals

The Leapfrog Group: www.leapfroggroup.org

The Picker Institute: http://pickerinstitute.org/

Planetree: www.planetree.org

HCAHPS: Hospital Care Quality Information from the Consumer Perspective:
www.hcahps.org

Consumer Assessment of Healthcare Providers and Systems Program:
www.cahps.ahrq.gov

UNDERSTANDING THE ROLE OF POLICY IN PROMOTING SYSTEM CHANGE

Learning Objectives

After completing this chapter you should be able to:

- define selected types of health policy;
- describe the role of quality oversight organizations;
- appreciate how public and private policy may fuel system change at the organizational, community, and national levels;
- analyze the role of quality reporting in system improvement; and
- identify resources to maintain current knowledge about policy changes, new initiatives, and updates on current initiatives.

The most visible or well-known topics of healthcare policy tend to be those related to funding, payment, and access. Examples include Titles XVIII and XIX, the Social Security Act Amendments of 1965 that created Medicare and Medicaid; the Balanced Budget Act of 1997 that created the State Children's Health Insurance Program (SCHIP); and the Patient Protection and Affordable Care Act signed into law in 2010 that aims to expand access to health insurance coverage in the United States. Public policy also plays an integral role in ensuring the quality of many other aspects of healthcare services.

Policies that control water, air, and food quality and, in turn, their respective effects on preventing disease in populations are fundamental to public health practice. Public policy also plays a role in promoting quality in healthcare services. Physicians, nurses, nurse practitioners, pharmacists, and other care providers require licenses to practice their professions and are guided by the statutes and rules outlined in the professional practice acts and occupational licensing bodies of their respective states. A physician's office may display evidence of professional credentials such as diplomas and board certification. Likewise, one will find evidence of the office's organizational credentials in the form of business licenses or accreditations posted visibly for customers, patients, and visitors. The ramped sidewalk to the front door of a health facility and tiny Braille numbers on the elevator buttons are design features influenced by the Americans with Disabilities Act. Sprinklers in the ceilings, signs labeled "fire exit," and special doors designed to close automatically fulfill building codes and fire safety requirements. Inappropriate or excessive radiation exposure to patients and healthcare personnel during diagnostic exams is prevented through meeting Occupational Safety and Health Administration requirements. The safety and efficacy of medications are investigated by the US Food and Drug Administration before release for patient use.

Within the context of Donabedian's model for measuring quality (see Chapter 1), policy initiatives have historically targeted the quality of the *structural elements* of the healthcare delivery system, such as people, physical facilities, equipment, and drugs. Outcome measures, such as infant mortality rates and life expectancy, and aggregate process measures, such as immunization rates, have been collected for many years by the public health infrastructure at the state, national, and international levels. Current health quality policy initiatives target outcomes and processes at the organization, provider, and population levels.

This chapter discusses the increasingly important role of public and private policies on healthcare quality by providing a brief overview of health policy concepts, explaining the role of quality oversight bodies, and introducing several healthcare quality initiatives that demonstrate the use of public and private policy to drive system change and improvement.

Health Policy: An Overview

The US government serves the following generic purposes: "to provide for those who cannot provide for themselves, to supply social and public goods, to regulate the market, and to instill trust and accountability" (Tang, Eisenberg, and Meyer 2004, 48). To accomplish these purposes, the government uses **public policy** or "authoritative decisions made in the legislative, executive, or judicial branches of government that are intended to direct or influence the actions, behaviors, or decisions of others" (Longest 2010, 5). **Private sector policy** complements public policy and guides governance and operations within a specific organization or as established by private organizations for the purpose of industry oversight (Longest 2010).

Regulatory policies are used to promote societal objectives in situations in which private markets do not function properly according to competitive market rules. These policies are designed to control economic forces, such as market entry, price, and quality, and to promote social aims, such as ensuring workplace safety and preventing spread of communicable disease (Longest 2010). **Allocative policies** are "designed to provide net benefits to some distinct group or class of individuals or organizations, at the expense of others, to ensure that public objectives are met" (Longest 2010, 13). For example, taxes provide pools of dollars that are redistributed to fund public

---

Public policy
"authoritative decisions made in the legislative, executive, or judicial branches of government that are intended to direct or influence the actions, behaviors, or decisions of others" (Longest 2010, 5)

Private sector policy
rules that guide governance and operations within a specific organization or as established by private organizations for the purpose of industry oversight (Longest 2010)

Regulatory policy
policy used to promote societal objectives in situations in which private markets do not function properly according to competitive market rules (Longest 2010)

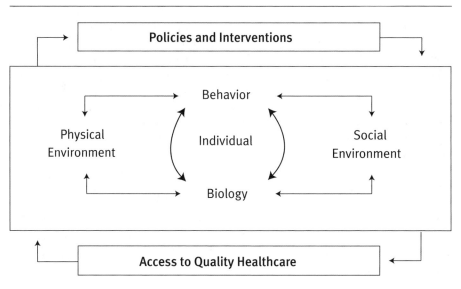

EXHIBIT 8.1

Healthy People 2010 Determinants of Health Model

Source: US Department of Health and Human Services (2000).

goods and services such as roads and law enforcement. **Health policies** are defined as policies that "pertain to health or influence the pursuit of health" (Longest 2010, 6). Health policies are crafted to influence health determinants, which in turn influence health. The Healthy People 2010 model, shown in Exhibit 8.1, illustrates the relationship among health policies, health determinants, and healthcare.

Health quality policy may be thought of as a subset within health policy. Government policies promote healthcare quality in a variety of ways. Tang, Eisenberg, and Meyer (2004, 47) list the government's 10 roles: "purchase health care, provide health care, ensure access to quality care for vulnerable populations, regulate health care markets, support acquisition of new knowledge, develop and evaluate health technologies and practices, monitor health care quality, inform health care decision makers, develop the health care workforce, and convene stakeholders from across the health care system." Within each of these functions are numerous strategies designed to accomplish the intended purpose.

Quality Oversight

A variety of federal, state, and local government agencies and private organizations assess, monitor, and oversee the quality of healthcare delivered by health plans, facilities, integrated delivery systems, and individual practitioners. Types of quality oversight organizations are summarized in Exhibit 8.2. The distinctions between three of these approaches are further described in Exhibit 8.3. **Licensure** is granted by a governmental body and represents

---

Allocative policies
policies "designed to provide net benefits to some distinct group or class of individuals or organizations, at the expense of others, to ensure that public objectives are met" (Longest 2010, 13)

Health policies
policies that "pertain to health or influence the pursuit of health" (Longest 2010, 6)

Licensure
granted by a governmental body and represents *minimum* standards

EXHIBIT 8.2

Types of
Healthcare
Quality
Oversight
Organizations
in the United
States

State Licensing Bodies. States, typically through their health departments, have long regulated healthcare delivery through the licensure of healthcare institutions such as hospitals, long-term care facilities, and home health agencies, as well as individual healthcare practitioners such as physicians and nurses. States also license, through their insurance and health departments, financial "risk-bearing entities," including both indemnity insurance products and those managed care products that perform the dual function of bearing risk (like an insurer) and arranging for or delivering healthcare services (like healthcare-providing entities).

Private Sector Accrediting Bodies. Accrediting bodies set standards for healthcare organizations and assess compliance with those standards. They also focus on the operation and effectiveness of internal quality improvement systems. In some areas, state and federal governments rely on or recognize private accreditation for purposes of ensuring compliance with licensure or regulatory requirements.

Medicare, Medicaid Compliance. For a healthcare entity to receive Medicare or Medicaid reimbursement, the entity must meet certain federally specified "Conditions of Participation" (COPs) or other standards. The US Health Care Financing Administration (HCFA)* promulgates COPs for hospitals, home health agencies, nursing facilities, hospices, ambulatory surgical centers, renal dialysis centers, rural health clinics, outpatient physical and occupation therapy, and rehabilitation facilities. HCFA also establishes standards for the participation of managed care organizations contracting under the Medicare program.

US Department of Labor. Oversight of certain aspects of employer-provided health plans is performed by the US Department of Labor. The Employee Retirement Income Security Act of 1974 sets minimum federal standards for group health plans maintained by private sector employers, unions, or jointly by employers and unions. The department oversees plan compliance with the following legal requirements of plan administration: reporting and disclosure of plan features and operations, fiduciary obligations for management of the plan and its assets, handling benefit claims, continuation coverage for workers who lose group health coverage, limitations on exclusions for pre-existing conditions, prohibitions on discrimination based on health status, renewability of group health coverage for employers, minimum hospital stays for childbirth, and parity of limits on mental health benefits.

Individual Certification and Credentialing Organizations. The American Board of Medical Specialties (an umbrella for 24 specialty boards) and the American Osteopathic Association have certification programs that designate certain medical providers as having completed specific training in a specialty and having passed examinations testing knowledge of that specialty. The Accreditation Council for Graduate Medical Education, sponsored by the American Medical Association and four other organizations, accredits nearly 7,700 residency programs in 1,600 medical institutions across the country. For nursing, the American Board of Nursing Specialties sets standards for the certification of

(continued)

nursing specialties. The largest numbers of nurses, both in generalist and specialist practice, are certified by the American Nurses Credentialing Center, based on practice standards established by the American Nurses Association.

EXHIBIT 8.2
(continued)

---

*Note: Since the publication of this report, the Health Care Financing Administration has been renamed the Centers for Medicare & Medicaid Services.

Source: President's Advisory Committee on Consumer Protection and Quality in the Health Care Industry (1998).

Licensure is a process by which a governmental authority grants permission to an individual practitioner or healthcare organization to operate or to engage in an occupation or profession. Licensure regulations are generally established to ensure that an organization or individual meets minimum standards to protect public health and safety. Licensure to individuals is usually granted after some form of examination or proof of education and may be renewed periodically through payment of a fee and/or proof of continuing education or professional competence.

EXHIBIT 8.3
Licensure,
Accreditation,
and
Certification

Organizational licensure is granted following an on-site inspection to determine if minimum health and safety standards have been met. Maintenance of licensure is an ongoing requirement for the healthcare organization to continue to operate and care for patients.

Accreditation is a formal process by which a recognized body, usually a non-governmental organization (NGO), assesses and recognizes that a healthcare organization meets applicable predetermined and published standards. Accreditation standards are usually regarded as optimal and achievable, and are designed to encourage continuous improvement efforts within accredited organizations. An accreditation decision about a specific healthcare organization is made following a periodic on-site evaluation by a team of peer reviewers, typically conducted every two to three years. Accreditation is often a voluntary process in which organizations choose to participate, rather than one required by law and regulation.

Standards [are] explicit, predetermined expectation[s] set by a competent authority that describes an organization's acceptable performance level. . . . Standards can develop from a variety of sources, from professional societies to panels of experts to research studies to regulations. Standards might also be organization-specific, such as those reflected in a hospital's clinical policies and procedures or clinical practice guidelines for the management of emergencies. Standards might evolve from a consensus of what are "best practices" given the current state of knowledge and technology.

Certification is a process by which an authorized body, either a governmental or non-governmental organization, evaluates and recognizes either an individual or an organization as meeting predetermined requirements or criteria.

(continued)

EXHIBIT 8.3
(continued)

Although the terms "accreditation" and "certification" are often used inter-changeably, accreditation usually applies only to organizations, while certification may apply to individuals as well as to organizations. When applied to individual practitioners, certification usually implies that the individual has received additional education and training and demonstrated competence in a specialty area beyond the minimum requirements set for licensure. An example of such a certification process is a physician who receives certification by a professional specialty board in the practice of obstetrics. When applied to an organization or part of an organization, such as the laboratory, certification usually implies that the organization has additional services, technology, or capacity beyond those found in similar organizations.

Source: Reprinted with permission from Rooney, A. L., and P. R. Ostenburg (1999). *Licensure, Accreditation, and Certification: Approaches to Health Service Quality.* Bethesda, MD, Quality Assurance Project, 3, 9. Retrieved 10/4/10 from www.who.int/management/quality/standards/en/index.html

Accreditation
a form of external quality review for health services organizations based on defining quality standards, assessing organizational compliance, and recognizing compliant organizations (Rooney and Ostenburg 1999)

Certification
a form of external quality review for health services professionals and organizations; when applied to individuals, it represents advanced education and competence; when applied to organizations, it represents meeting predetermined standards for a specialized service provided by the organization (Rooney and Ostenburg 1999)

minimum standards, while **accreditation** and **certification** are granted by non-governmental organizations and represent *optimal* standards or *advanced* education and competence.

The Joint Commission is a non-governmental accreditation organization for the following types of health services organizations: ambulatory care, behavioral health care, critical access hospitals, home care, hospitals, laboratory services, long-term care, and office-based surgery (The Joint Commission 2010a). The Joint Commission also offers disease-specific certification for organizations offering services for conditions such as chronic kidney disease, diabetes (inpatient), and stroke (The Joint Commission 2010a). The National Committee for Quality Assurance (NCQA) offers accreditation programs for health plans and related organizations and programs such as wellness and health promotion and disease management. The NCQA also offers a variety of certifications (NCQA 2010). After several years of development and testing, the Public Health Accreditation Board implemented the National Public Health Voluntary Accreditation Program, in 2011 (PHAB 2010). Additional accreditation organizations are listed in the Web Resources box.

Knowledge Acquisition

Public policy at the federal level creates formal structures and mechanisms for acquiring new knowledge so that public and private policymakers may make informed, evidence-based decisions about health quality policies. For example, the Agency for Healthcare Research and Quality (AHRQ) sponsors and conducts research and disseminates information to advance healthcare quality (see Exhibit 8.4).

The Centers for Medicare & Medicaid Services (CMS) supports local implementation of federal policies through its network of state-based Quality Improvement Organizations (Leavitt 2006, 2).

Mission: To support research designed to improve the quality, safety, efficiency, and effectiveness of healthcare for all Americans. The research sponsored, conducted, and disseminated by the Agency for Healthcare Research and Quality (AHRQ) provides information that helps people make better decisions about healthcare.

Created: December 1989 as the Agency for Health Care Policy and Research (AHCPR), a public health service agency in the US Department of Health and Human Services (HHS). Reporting to the HHS Secretary, the agency was reauthorized on December 6, 1999, as the Agency for Healthcare Research and Quality.

Sister agencies include the National Institutes of Health, the Centers for Disease Control and Prevention, the Food and Drug Administration, the Centers for Medicare & Medicaid Services, and the Health Resources and Services Administration.

Main functions: AHRQ sponsors and conducts research that provides evidence-based information on healthcare outcomes; quality; and cost, use, and access. The information helps healthcare decision makers—patients and clinicians, health system leaders, purchasers, and policymakers—make more informed decisions and improve the quality of healthcare services.

EXHIBIT 8.4
Agency for
Healthcare
Research and
Quality

Source: AHRQ (2008a).

The Medicare Quality Improvement Organization (QIO) Program (formerly referred to as the Medicare Utilization and Quality Control Peer Review Program) was created by statute in 1982 to improve quality and efficiency of services delivered to Medicare beneficiaries. In its first phase, which concluded in the early nineties, the Program sought to accomplish its mission through peer review of cases to identify instances in which professional standards were not met for purposes of initiating corrective actions. In the second phase, quality measurement and improvement became the predominant mode of Program operation.

This network serves the community of providers caring for Medicare beneficiaries through technical assistance, beneficiary advocacy, pilot programs, measurement, evaluation, and research. The three-year QIO contract cycle is designed to align the work of the QIOs with CMS strategic initiatives.

Public Policy Promoting Systems Change

The contemporary view of quality management expands the concept of "customer" to include stakeholders and markets in which the organization operates (see Chapter 1). The quality oversight organizations are vital stakeholders of health services organizations. Their standards, regulations, and conditions of participation are increasingly being used to drive system change and improve quality of care and services. Details on specific laws and regulations, and impact of healthcare quality, may be found in other texts dedicated to health policy. In this section, a few key examples are presented that illustrate the role of policy in system improvement. Background on the evolution of these initiatives is also provided so readers may appreciate the influence of history on the current healthcare quality landscape.

Transparency—Centers for Medicare & Medicaid Services

Public disclosure or "transparency" has proven to be an effective strategy to reduce risk for consumers and promote accountability of businesses in other industries. For example, "in 1986 Congress passed a new law requiring manufacturers to reveal to the public their toxic releases in standardized form, chemical by chemical and factory by factory" (Graham 2002). Subsequently, the amount of toxic chemicals that manufacturers released into the environment declined by 46 percent between the years 1988 and 1999. Public disclosure has a long history in the United States. The Securities and Exchange Acts passed in the 1930s required publicly traded companies to publish earnings data. These two examples illustrate the power of information as a "regulatory mechanism" (Graham 2002).

In 1987, the Health Care Financing Agency (HCFA), now known as the Centers for Medicare & Medicaid Services or CMS, produced its first annual report of "observed hospital-specific mortality rates for Medicare acute care hospitals" (Cleves and Golden 1996, 40). In the early description of the HCFA Effectiveness Initiative, William Roper, the director of HCFA at the time, explains why this type of effort must be undertaken by the federal agency. He states that "information about the effectiveness of particular services provides a public good. . . . [H]owever, because the benefit of better information accrues to the public at large, not just to those collecting it, the market system may not ensure adequate investment in the necessary research and data collection" (Roper et al. 1988, 1197).

While healthcare differs from securities and environmental pollution, using information to reduce risk to healthcare consumers has potential in a market economy. To understand the potential value of transparency in healthcare, it helps to understand the risks US healthcare consumers face:

- "Evidence on the variations in medical care across geographic regions in the United States suggests that as much as 30 percent of spending reflects medical care of uncertain or questionable value. Overall, the Institute of Medicine has estimated that less than 50 percent of treatments delivered today are supported by evidence" (Tunis, Benner, and McClellan 2010, 1963).

- In the United States, 5 to 10 percent of patients hospitalized develop healthcare-associated infections (HAIs) and each year 100,000 people die as a result of an HAI (Yokoe and Classen 2008, S3).
- Five preventable hospital-acquired complications (decubitus ulcers, postoperative bleeding, postoperative pulmonary embolism/deep vein thrombosis, postoperative infection, and iatrogenic pneumothorax) cost Medicare over $300 million annually, yet "these extra payments cover less than a third of the extra costs incurred by hospitals in treating these adverse events" (Zhan et al. 2006).
- In 2009, only 72 percent of children ages 19 to 35 months were appropriately immunized (Kaiser Family Foundation 2011).

The goal of the early efforts of HCFA's Effectiveness Initiative was to produce "better information to guide the decisions of physicians, patients, and the agency, thus improving outcomes and the quality of care" (Roper et al. 1988, 1198). The initiative consisted of the following components:

> First . . . data from the Medicare systems of claims processing and peer review [are being used] to monitor trends and assess the effectiveness of specific interventions. . . . Second, plans for a data resource center are being developed and files of Medicare data are being made available for appropriate research by private persons and organizations. . . . Third, clinical research is being funded, both intramurally and extramurally, that will examine the appropriateness and effectiveness of various procedures. . . . Finally, the methods of conducting research on effectiveness are being improved and the data bases expanded. (Roper et al. 1988, 1198)

This strategy set the stage for using federal policy to systematically develop and implement expectations, requirements, methodology, and infrastructure to collect, publish, and disseminate quality performance data measuring beneficiaries' quality of care. Performance data are now readily available to the public via the CMS website (www.cms.gov/center/quality.asp). The mortality data reports were discontinued in 1994 and the focus turned to high-volume, high-cost clinical conditions.

Between 1997 and 1999, HCFA collected quality process measures on acute myocardial infarction (AMI), breast cancer, diabetes mellitus, congestive heart failure (CHF), pneumonia, and stroke. Noteworthy about the study was that unlike the mortality data derived from administrative claims data, these data were abstracted directly from the patients' clinical records. The aim was not only to compare effectiveness of care on a national level but also to establish a reliable methodology for collecting quality process measures with "strong scientific evidence and professional consensus that the process of care either directly improves outcomes or is a necessary step in a chain of care that does so" (Jencks et al. 2000, 1670). Study results documented performance in the 24 clinical process measures (Jencks et al. 2000).

The performance data collection was repeated between 2000 and 2001 and compared to the 1997–1999 baseline. This follow-up study, published in 2003, showed improved performance in 22 of 24 of the original measures (Jencks, Huff, and Cuerdon 2003). In 2003, CMS established the voluntary reporting initiative, where eligible hospitals could voluntarily report their performance on quality indicators in the three conditions of AMI, CHF, and community-acquired pneumonia (CAP). In 2005, hospital-specific results were posted on the US Department of Health and Human Services website called "Hospital Compare" for public access and review.

Since that time, the number and type of quality measures for hospitals have continued to grow each year. For fiscal year 2011, CMS tracks 46 quality measures including clinical process measures in AMI, CHF, CAP, and surgical care; the Hospital Consumer Assessment of Health Providers and Systems (HCAHPS); and recently introduced outcome indicators (CMS 2010b, 2010c).

Providers in most settings of care for Medicare beneficiaries must report quality measures. In addition to the Hospital Compare website, the public has access to Nursing Home Compare, Home Health Compare, and Dialysis Facility Compare. Please refer to the Web Resources box for more information about these initiatives.

Financial Incentives—Centers for Medicare & Medicaid Services

To induce participation in voluntary reporting, Section 501(b) of the Medicare Prescription Drug, Improvement, and Modernization Act (MMA) of 2003 established the Reporting Hospital Quality Data for Annual Payment Update (RHQDAPU) initiative, which "authorized CMS to pay hospitals that successfully report designated quality measures a higher annual update to their payment rates. Initially, the MMA provided for a 0.4-percent reduction in the annual market basket (the measure of inflation in costs of goods and services used by hospitals in treating Medicare patients) update for hospitals that did not successfully report" (CMS 2010d). The Deficit Reduction Act of 2005 increased the reduction in the market basket update for non-reporting hospitals from 0.4 percent to 2 percent. In 2006, the voluntary reporting initiative for HCAHPS began, and in 2008 HCAHPS reporting was incorporated into the RHQDAPU. By "FY 2009, 96 percent of hospitals participated successfully in the reporting program and received the full market basket update for FY 2010" (CMS 2010d).

The implementation of the prospective payment system by CMS in the 1980s focused on containing the increasing costs of hospital care. The transparency initiatives described previously focused on defining, documenting, and reporting quality of care to the public. The next phase of CMS quality policy focuses on **value**, a ratio of quality to cost (value = quality / cost). The Deficit Reduction Act of 2005 (DRA) established the Hospital-Acquired Conditions and Present on Admission Indicator Reporting (HAC & POA)

Value
ratio of quality to cost (value = quality / cost)

initiative, which states, "For discharges occurring on or after October 1, 2008, IPPS hospitals will not receive additional payment for cases when one of the selected conditions is acquired during hospitalization (i.e., was not present on admission). The case would be paid as though the secondary diagnosis were not present" (CMS 2010e, 1).

Consider the historical role of clinical complications and hospital payment. If a surgical sponge was accidently left inside the patient after surgery and the patient required another surgery to remove it, both surgeries were billed to the payer. The HAC & POA initiative is based on the principle that CMS will not pay for complications that should not have occurred in the first place. The following criteria led to a list of conditions, also referred to as "never events" (CMS 2010e, 1); conditions which

- are high-cost or high-volume or both,
- result in the assignment of a case to an MS-DRG that has a higher payment when present as a secondary diagnosis, and
- could reasonably have been prevented through the application of evidence-based guidelines.

A continued focus on value is the theme of contemporary healthcare quality policy at the federal level. Value is now the foundational criterion upon which beneficiary services are purchased (CMS 2010f). Establishment of the Center for Medicare and Medicaid Innovation as a provision of the Patient Protection and Affordable Care Act of 2010 guarantees ongoing research, demonstration projects, and initiatives to advance CMS toward value-based purchasing. The purpose of the center "is to test innovative payment and delivery system models that show important promise for maintaining or improving the quality of care in Medicare, Medicaid, and the Children's Health Insurance Program (CHIP)" (Guterman et al. 2010, 1188).

Private Policy Promoting Systems Change

Parallel to the development of quality reporting initiatives by CMS, The Joint Commission initiated its ORYX initiative for hospital quality indicators (Chassin et al. 2010). The Joint Commission and CMS recognize the importance of a unified approach between public-policy and private-policy initiatives and have actively collaborated to align quality reporting measures and methodologies. As stated in the *Specifications Manual for National Hospital Inpatient Quality Measures* (The Joint Commission and CMS 2010):

> Since November of 2003, CMS and The Joint Commission have worked to precisely and completely align these common measures so that they are identical. This resulted in the creation of one common set of measure specifications. . . . The goal is to minimize data

collection efforts for these common measures and focus efforts on the use of data to improve the healthcare delivery process.

Through its conditions for participation and conditions for coverage, CMS (2010a) "also ensures that the standards of accrediting organizations recognized by CMS (through a process called 'deeming') meet or exceed Medicare standards." The combined quality requirements of public and private stakeholders are aimed at accelerating the pace of system improvement.

Accreditation Approach: The Joint Commission

The Joint Commission realized the limitations of the traditional accreditation process and has aggressively introduced changes that require health services organizations to move along the quality continuum if they are to meet accreditation requirements. Started in 1999 and officially launched in 2004, The Joint Commission's Shared Visions—New Pathways accreditation process is described as "a paradigm shift from a process focused on survey preparation to one of continuous systematic and operational improvement by focusing to a greater extent on the provision of safe, high quality care, treatment and services" (The Joint Commission and Joint Commission Resources 2004, 1).

This redesigned approach to accreditation includes revised and streamlined accreditation standards, use of organizational data to tailor the accreditation process to the organization's specific needs and patient population, a focus on continuous compliance by combining unannounced on-site surveys with online compliance documentation, enhanced electronic communication between The Joint Commission and health services organizations, and the introduction of the tracer methodology for on-site surveys, which emphasizes the interrelatedness of care process and standards throughout the organization (Joint Commission Resources 2003; The Joint Commission 2010b).

In the past, surveyors relied on document review (i.e., policies, procedures, administrative records, and patients' clinical records) to determine an organization's compliance with Joint Commission standards. The redesigned process focuses on direct observation and discussions with care providers, other frontline employees, and patients, and real-time document review as the primary sources of information.

The Joint Commission has also incorporated an on-site survey process called the **tracer methodology**, which provides the opportunity to examine the depth and breadth of an organization's quality and safety efforts. For example, infection control, medication management, data use, and environment of care are so important to patient quality and safety that The Joint Commission has designated them as priority areas for in-depth evaluation within and across departments in the organization. In a **system tracer**, the surveyor examines the multiple processes, systems, and structures that make up these priority areas. For example, a system tracer for medication management would include processes for how an organization selects, stores, orders, dispenses, and administers

---

Tracer methodology
The Joint Commission's on-site survey method that provides the opportunity to examine the depth and breadth of an organization's quality and safety efforts

---

System tracer
The Joint Commission's in-depth examination of the multiple processes, systems, and structures that make up the priority areas such as infection control, medication management, data use, and environment of care

medications as well as how the providers evaluate the effectiveness of a drug therapy and identify, track, and prevent adverse drug events. The system tracer methodology takes into account the "set of components that work together toward a common goal . . . and how well the organization's systems function. This approach addresses the interrelationships of the many elements that go into delivering safe, high-quality care and translates standards compliance issues into potential organizational vulnerabilities" (Cockshut-Miller 2004, 14). Exhibit 8.5 shows a schematic of the system tracer approach.

System Tracer

The surveyor "traces" the elements of the system.

EXHIBIT 8.5

System and Individual Tracers

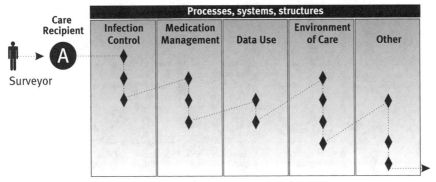

Individual Tracer

The surveyor "traces" the course of care provided to the recipient.

♦ = Standards evaluation opportunities related to individual care recipient experiences across multiple functions (for example, dispensing and administration in medication management).

Source: © Joint Commission Resources: *Tracer Methodology: Tips and Strategies for Continuous Systems Improvement.* Oakbrook Terrace, IL: Joint Commission on Accreditation of Healthcare Organizations, 2004, 5–6. Reprinted with permission.

Individual tracer
The Joint Commission's in-depth examination that follows a patient's experience within the organization

While a system tracer follows one of the priority areas throughout the organization, an **individual tracer** follows a patient's experience within the organization. Surveyors evaluate whether the delivery of care is executed in a manner that complies with standards within the context of the patient's progression through the episode of care. Based on the data collected about the organization before the survey, a patient condition is selected.

When the surveyors arrive on site, an actual patient is chosen from the current patient census. Questions are posed to staff currently caring for this patient and to staff in all of the other departments who have interacted or may interact with this patient during her current stay or visit. "Just as an individual's care encompass[es] several standards at one time, surveyors focus on a number of related processes of care rather than just one process. . . . For example, re-assessment, nutrition, medical equipment risks, and caregiver competencies might all be considered when tracing the care of a resident in a long-term-care facility. . . . [U]nder the new accreditation process, it is not as important for staff to know what the . . . standard is, but rather to know how they provide safe, high-quality care, treatment and services to individuals" (The Joint Commission and Joint Commission Resources 2004, 10). Exhibit 8.6 shows a schematic of an individual tracer. The exhibit illustrates the complementary nature of the two types of tracers used in the survey process and how, when used together, they provide a comprehensive picture of the organization's systems approach to quality and safety.

EXHIBIT 8.6
Combined System and Individual Tracer

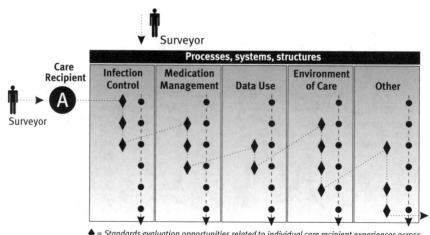

♦ = Standards evaluation opportunities related to individual care recipient experiences across multiple functions (for example, dispensing and administration in medication management).

Note: Dashed vertical arrows reflect standards evaluation opportunities related to exploration of the design of a system and the dots represent any given elements of a system.

Source: © Joint Commission Resources: *Tracer Methodology: Tips and Strategies for Continuous Systems Improvement*. Oakbrook Terrace, IL: Joint Commission on Accreditation of Healthcare Organizations, 2004, 5–6. Reprinted with permission.

Lessons for Managers

Early efforts by hospitals to fulfill the quality reporting requirements appeared to have been segmented according to clinical conditions (i.e., AMI, heart failure, and community-acquired pneumonia), which resulted in variable performance across conditions (Jha et al. 2005). In other words, care may have improved for cardiac patients, but not for patients with pneumonia; care may have improved for patients with the three conditions being measured, but not necessarily for all patients receiving care within the hospital.

Lessons from epidemiology regarding etiology provide insights into how CMS quality-reporting requirements may be used to improve not only select conditions, but the organizational system as a whole. When considering the underlying causes of disease, Rose (2001, 428) discusses the "two kinds of etiology question(s). The first seeks the cause of cases and the second seeks the cause of incidence. 'Why do some individuals have hypertension?' is quite a different question from 'Why do some populations have much hypertension whilst in others it is rare?' The answers require different kinds of study and they have different answers."

Just as in the etiology of disease, the questions about etiology may be applied to understanding systemic structure within the context of the iceberg metaphor. For example, consider the levels of questions about one of the CMS quality indicators for AMI in Exhibit 8.7.

As the number of required quality indicators for reporting grows, patterns in the indicators become more visible. Exhibit 8.8 shows an example of how patterns may be identified by grouping similar indicators and how those patterns may lead to system structure questions.

Level	Question	Underlying Cause	
Event/individual case question	Why didn't *this patient* with an AMI receive aspirin on admission to the emergency department (ED)?	The department was extremely busy and under-staffed that day. The aspirin was ordered but not given.	**EXHIBIT 8.7** Levels of Questions About CMS Quality Indicators
Patterns/process-level question	Why don't *patients admitted to this ED* with AMI consistently receive aspirin on arrival to the ED?	Emergency physician services are outsourced to a private group. Each physician has her own set of "standing orders."	
Systemic structure/incidence within a population-level question	Why isn't evidence-based care consistently practiced at this hospital?	Unless a problem arises, the hospital CEO and COO operate from a "hands off" philosophy when it comes to medical care and decisions.	

EXHIBIT 8.8

Forming
System
Structure
Questions by
Identifying
Patterns and
Grouping
Indicators

Event → (individual indicator)	Patterns → (like indicators)	Systemic Structure Questions
Process indicators for Group 1		
Preoperative antibiotics	Patients at risk for a surgical infection	How are "at risk" patients identified?
Treatment for DVT/PE	Patients at risk for a DVT/PE	
Pneumococcal vaccine	Patients at risk for developing flu and subsequent respiratory illness/complications	Once identified, how are care processes "activated" to prevent complications associated with the risk?
HAC/POA indicators		
Falls with injury	Patients at risk for falls	
Pressure ulcer stage III/IV	Patients at risk for pressure ulcers	How are the risks documented on admission and communicated throughout the episode of care?
Catheter-associated UTI	Patients at risk for infections	
Vascular catheter–associated infection		
Process indicators for Group 2		
Smoking cessation Advice/counseling	Preparing for discharge	How are activities related to transition from an inpatient episode to the next level of care defined?
Aspirin at discharge		
Beta blocker at discharge		
Heart failure discharge instructions		How are activities that assist in patient self-management and reducing acute exacerbation of a chronic condition defined and implemented during an inpatient episode of care?
Children and their caregivers receiving a Home Management Plan of Care document while hospitalized for asthma		

As Chapter 1 describes, organizational effectiveness aims to combine the knowledge of management and quality to understand and improve the organization. Similarly, an understanding of systemic structure helps managers target system change that guides improving processes (patterns), which in turn improve care to the individual patient (events). In other words, the direction of managerial actions follows the arrows shown in Exhibit 8.9.

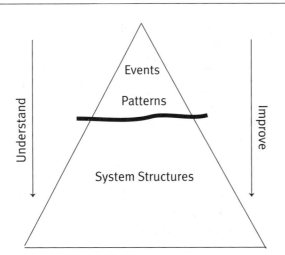

EXHIBIT 8.9
The Iceberg
Metaphor and
Organizational
Effectiveness

Private healthcare policy, such as Joint Commission accreditation requirements, has and will likely continue to address system structures that move organizations as systems along the quality continuum. Some describe the least mature end of the quality continuum as "little q" and the mature end as "big Q" (Juran 1989). In little q, quality is the concern of specialists; in big Q, quality is the concern of everyone. Consider the areas of risks and patient safety. Evolving Joint Commission standards have expanded the accountability for identifying and managing patient and organizational risks from the confines of the risk management department to requirements integrated throughout the various standards groups. The following examples are from the 2010 hospital standards (The Joint Commission 2010d; Kelly 2009d).

- Leadership: LD.01.04.01 A chief executive manages the hospital. EP (elements of performance): The chief executive provides for the following: *Physical and financial assets.*
- Environment of Care: EC.02.03.01 The hospital manages fire *risks.*
- Medication Management: MM.01.01.03 The hospital safely manages *high-alert and hazardous medications.*
- Information Management: IM.02.01.03 The hospital maintains the *security and integrity of health information.*
- Patient Care: PC.03.01.03 The hospital provides the patient with care before initiating operative or other *high-risk procedures,* including those that require the administration of deep sedation or anesthesia.
- National Patient Safety Goal 7: Reduce the *risk* of healthcare-associated infection.

National healthcare quality policy in the public domain is evolving from a focus on individual conditions and facilities to the collective interrelationships of multiple organizations involved in providing health services. At the time of this writing, several CMS demonstration projects are under way that link quality initiatives along the continuum of care and to populations of beneficiaries.

Healthcare quality policy continues to evolve with the passage of the Patient Protection and Affordable Care Act of 2010. Title III of the act, "Improving the Quality and Efficiency of Health Care," contains numerous provisions that target systemic structures, at the individual, organizational, professional, and community levels, that have historically impeded system improvement (Patient Protection and Affordable Care Act of 2010).

According to *Improving America's Hospitals: The Joint Commission's Annual Report on Quality and Safety*, progress is being made in improving care, as reflected in the publicly reported indicators (The Joint Commission 2010c).

> Nineteen measures have been followed for eight years (2002–2009) and 11 more have been followed from five to two years. The magnitude of improvement on the individual accountability measures had a median value of 8.6 percent for 23 of the 24 measures and ranged from –0.5 percent (for a measure with two years of reporting experience) to +62.6 percent (for one measure with eight years of reporting experience). While there were differing amounts of improvement over the measures, all but one measure showed improvement over the range of reporting experience. That measure—the surgical care measure for beta-blocker patients who received beta-blocker perioperatively—had only two years of reporting experience. With that one exception, all of the measures consistently showed year-over-year improvement.

Summary

Public and private policy bodies have increasingly used their influence as stakeholders to fuel the quality agenda in healthcare services. This chapter discusses the role of quality oversight organizations and introduces key national policy initiatives that target system change. These initiatives include the CMS initiatives around transparency, quality reporting, and incentives. The redesign of The Joint Commission's accreditation approach is also discussed. The examples are discussed within the context of the iceberg metaphor to illustrate how public and private policy can serve as an impetus for system change. Because of the dynamic and rapidly changing nature of healthcare quality policy, especially with the passing of the Patient Protection and Affordable Care Act of 2010, readers are encouraged to review the accompanying Internet resources as a means to keep current on changes, new initiatives, and plans for the future.

Exercise

Objective: To become familiar with the CMS quality initiatives.

Instructions:

- Based on your work setting or an area of interest, select and explore one of the CMS quality initiatives (e.g., hospitals, home health, nursing home, dialysis, physician) at www.cms.hhs.gov/quality.
- Answer the following questions in reference to the selected resource:
  a. In two to three paragraphs, describe the contents of this resource and its relationship to healthcare quality.
  b. Describe how the information contained on this site may be used in the organizational setting you studied.
  c. Choose, analyze, and interpret one data set contained in this resource.

Companion Readings

Centers for Medicare & Medicaid Services (CMS). 2010. "Roadmap for Quality Measurement in the Traditional Medicare Fee-for-Service Program." [Online information; retrieved 4/5/11.] www.cms.gov/center/quality.asp

Guterman, S., K. Davis, K. Stremikis, and H. Drake. 2010. "Innovation in Medicare and Medicaid Will Be Central to Health Reform's Success." *Health Affairs* 29 (6): 1188–93.

National Quality Forum. 2010. "The Power of Safety: State Reporting Provides Lessons in Reducing Harm, Improving Care." [Online article.] www.qualityforum.org/Publications/2010/06/The_Power_of_Safety_State_Reporting_Provides_Lessons_in_Reducing_Harm,_Improving_Care.aspx

Roper, W. L., W. Winkenwerder, G. M. Hackbarth, and H. Krakauer. 1988. "Effectiveness in Health Care: An Initiative to Evaluate and Improve Medical Practice." *New England Journal of Medicine* 319: 1197–202.

Skyve, P. M. 2009. "Leadership in Healthcare Organizations: A Guide to Joint Commission Leadership Standards." A Governance Institute Whitepaper. [Online whitepaper.] www.jointcommission.org/NR/rdonlyres/48366FFD-DB16-4C91-98F3-46C552A18D2A/0/WP_Leadership_Standards.pdf

Web Resources

Accreditation

Accreditation Council for Pharmacy Education (ACPE): www.acpe-accredit.org/
Accreditation Association for Ambulatory Health Care (AAAHC):
    www.aaahc.org
Accreditation Council for Graduate Medical Education (ACGME):
    www.acgme.org
College of American Pathologists (CAP): www.cap.org
Commission on Accreditation of Rehabilitation Facilities (CARF): www.carf.org
Commission on Collegiate Nursing Education (CCNE):
    www.aacn.nche.edu/Accreditation/index.htm
Community Health Accreditation Program (CHAP): www.chapinc.org
National Committee for Quality Assurance (NCQA): www.ncqa.org
National League for Nursing Accrediting Commission, Inc. (NLNAC):
    www.nlnac.org/home.htm
National Public Health Performance Standards Program (NPHPSP):
    www.cdc.gov/od/ocphp/nphpsp/index.htm
Public Health Accreditation Board (PHAB): www.phaboard.org
The Joint Commission: www.jointcommission.org
URAC (formerly the Utilization Review Accreditation Commission):
    www.urac.org

Reports

Quality Interagency Coordination Task Force ("Doing What Counts for
    Patient Safety: Federal Actions to Reduce Medical Errors and Their
    Impact"): www.quic.gov/report/toc.htm
CMS Quality of Care Center (with links to compare websites):
    www.cms.gov/center/quality.asp

Informing Policymakers

Agency for Healthcare Research and Quality: www.ahrq.gov/
Institute of Medicine: www.iom.edu/
National Quality Forum: www.qualityforum.org/
Quality Improvement Organization Directory:
    www.qualitynet.org/dcs/ContentServer?pagename=Medqic/
    MQGeneralPage/GeneralPageTemplate&name=QIO%20Listings

Patient Protection and Affordable Care Act of 2010

Healthcare.gov: www.healthcare.gov
The Henry J. Kaiser Family Foundation Health Reform Source:
    healthreform.kff.org/

IMPROVING PROCESSES
AND IMPLEMENTING IMPROVEMENTS

Learning Objectives

After completing this chapter you should be able to:

- compare and contrast managerial approaches used for systematic improvement;
- differentiate how, when, and why to use common improvement tools; and
- explain a framework for implementing improvements in complex systems and the system lessons upon which the framework is based.

An employee is faced with choosing a new primary care physician when her employer changes health plans. This employee makes a list of the characteristics she wants in a physician (e.g., board certified) and in the physician's office (e.g., close to work). She asks fellow employees and friends if they know any of the physicians listed in the health plan handbook and what they think of their care experiences. She then selects a physician and makes an appointment for an annual physical. After her first experience with the new physician, she decides that the physician and the office staff meet her criteria and that she will continue to use the physician as her primary care physician.

She *planned* how to select a physician; *collected data* about her options; *compared* the various options against her criteria; *tested* her first choice; and, based on her impressions and experiences, *decided* to keep her first choice as her primary care physician. Although this employee may not have realized it, the continuous-improvement approach used in her organization had "rubbed off" on her so that she automatically used the same systematic process for deciding what to do when faced with a personal problem or decision.

In the clinical setting, clinical providers use the scientific method and the evidence-based process (JAMA 2010) to systematically solve problems. For example, a patient presents with a complaint. The provider gathers subjective data (what the patient tells him) and objective data (e.g., vital signs, physical exam, diagnostic tests); diagnoses the problem based on the patient data; devises a patient plan according to the diagnosis; implements the plan; evaluates the patient's response (e.g., collects additional subjective and objective data and compares to previous data); and revises the plan as needed. When clinical professionals use the scientific method in decision making, it is often referred to as "professional judgment" (Facione et al. 2002). Likewise, managerial professional judgment may be described by the concept of *critical thinking*.

This chapter presents systematic improvement approaches to aid managers in developing their improvement thinking, tools to assist managers in better understanding process problems and in designing process improvements, and an implementation framework to enable managers to implement change within complex systems.

Systematic Critical Thinking in Designing Improvements

Critical thinking is also essential within the management domain.

> Everyone thinks; it is our nature to do so. But much of our thinking, left to itself, is biased, distorted, partial, uninformed or downright prejudiced. Yet the quality of our life and that of what we produce, make, or build depends precisely on the quality of our thought. Shoddy thinking is costly, both in money and in quality of life. Excellence in thought, however, must be systematically cultivated. (Critical Thinking Community 2010)

Critical thinking
"the art of analyzing and evaluating thinking with a view to improving it" (Critical Thinking Community 2010)

The broader the scope of responsibility managers have in a health services organization, the greater the imperative to develop, cultivate, and refine their critical thinking skills. **Critical thinking** is essential if managers are to be effective stewards of limited human resources, financial resources, and the patients' lives and health that are entrusted to their organizations or their community. Within the context of quality management, managers have numerous approaches and tools to guide and maximize their critical thinking skills.

Continuous Improvement Cycle

Shewhart cycle
(also referred to as the PDCA cycle) consists of four continuous steps: plan, do, check/study, and act

Applying critical thinking to a problem or performance gap is illustrated by the TQM principle of continuous improvement (see Chapter 1). The employee in this chapter's opening example used an adaptation of what is referred to in the quality improvement literature as the Shewhart cycle or Deming Wheel (Exhibit 9.1).

Originating from industrial applications of quality improvement, the **Shewhart cycle** (also referred to as the PDCA cycle) consists of four steps: planning, doing, checking or studying, and acting. The steps are linked to

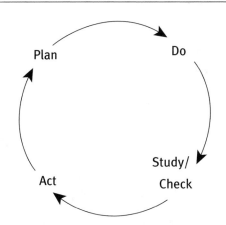

EXHIBIT 9.1
Shewhart Cycle

Source: From Deming, W. E. 2000. *Out of the Crisis,* p. 88. Cambridge, MA: The MIT Press. © MIT Press.

represent the cyclical nature of the approach. The steps in this systematic and continuous approach to improvement are (ASQ 2010b):

- Plan: Identify an opportunity and plan for change.
- Do: Implement the change on a small scale.
- Check or Study: Use data to analyze the results of the change and determine whether it made a difference.
- Act: If the change was successful, implement it on a wider scale and continuously assess your results. If the change did not work, begin the cycle again.

The improvement model (IHI 2011) adds the following three questions before applying the PDCA cycle to a problem or performance gap:

1. What are we trying to accomplish?
2. How will we know that a change is an improvement?
3. What change can we make that will result in an improvement?

Employees at all levels of an organization—from entry level to the executive suite—may use this simple continuous improvement thought process to promote critical problem solving in the work setting.

Six Sigma DMAIC

Another example of applying critical thinking in a systematic way to improve a problem is the **Six Sigma DMAIC** methodology. These steps, illustrated in Exhibit 9.2, may be viewed as an ongoing process similar to the PDCA cycle.

Six Sigma DMAIC
define, measure, analyze, improve, control

EXHIBIT 9.2
Six Sigma
DMAIC

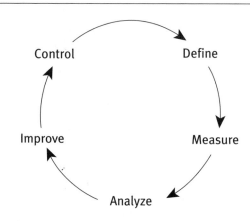

The DMAIC cycle adds more definition to the PDCA cycle, explicitly focuses improvement on root causes, and addresses ongoing evaluation and control. The steps are defined as (ASQ 2010c):

- Define a problem or improvement opportunity.
- Measure process performance.
- Analyze the process to determine the root causes of poor performance; determine whether the process can be improved or should be redesigned.
- Improve the process by attacking root causes.
- Control the improved process to hold the gains.

EXHIBIT 9.3
Performance
Management
Cycle

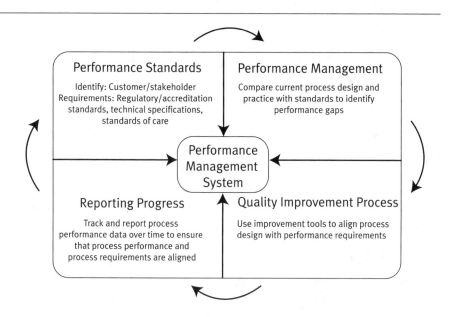

Source: Adapted with permission from The Public Health Foundation "From Silos to Systems," p. 12.

Performance Management Cycle

When the scope of application of the previous improvement cycles is expanded from a single process to the manager's domain of responsibility (i.e., department, program, or organization), the manager is best served by the performance management cycle shown in Exhibit 9.3. The **performance management cycle** links performance standards, performance measurement, performance improvement, and reporting progress in an ongoing cycle. This perspective emphasizes the need to continuously review, evaluate, and integrate changing customer, stakeholder, and regulatory requirements (see Chapter 7).

Performance management cycle links the performance standards, performance measurement, performance improvement, and reporting progress in an ongoing cycle

Process Improvement Tools

Document the Process

Some of the most valuable improvement tools are those that help managers and teams better understand work processes. Often a process is followed because "that is how we have always done it" or because a certain way of doing things has simply evolved over time. Before a process can be improved, it must be understood. The tools described in this section help managers and teams understand processes by documenting the steps involved.

According to the American Society for Quality, a **process** is "an organized group of related activities that work together to transform one or more kinds of input into outputs that are of value to the customer" (ASQ 2002). This definition suggests the following key features of a process (ASQ 2010d, italics added):

Process "an organized group of related activities that work together to transform one or more kinds of input into outputs that are of value to the customer" (ASQ 2002)

- A process is a *group of activities*, not just one.
- The activities that make up a process are not random or ad hoc; they are *related and organized*.
- All the activities in a process must work together toward a *common goal*.
- Processes exist to create *results your customers care about*.

A **process flowchart** is a picture of the sequence of steps in a process. Types of activities are represented by different-shaped symbols. An oval indicates the start and end of the process, a rectangle indicates a process action step, and a diamond indicates a decision that must be made in the process. Depending on the decision, the process follows different paths. A simple process flowchart is illustrated in Exhibit 9.4. Clinical providers may already be familiar with this tool, as many clinical algorithms and guidelines are communicated using process flowcharts. Other specialties such as laboratory, radiology, and information systems professionals may also be familiar with this tool as more complex versions of a process flowchart are

Process flowchart a picture of the sequence of steps in a process

EXHIBIT 9.4

Simple Process
Flowchart

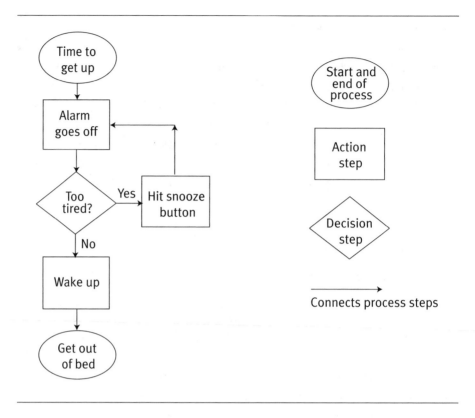

**Deployment
flowchart**
process flowchart
diagram that
includes and dis-
tinguishes who
is responsible for
which steps of the
process

used to document technical standard operating procedures (SOPs) or data and information flow.

Sometimes many individuals, departments, or organizations are involved in carrying out different steps of a single process. In this case a **deployment flowchart** (vertical flowchart) or "swim lanes" chart (horizontal flowchart) is used to distinguish who is responsible for which steps of the process. Efforts to improve coordination of process steps may be enhanced by identifying, documenting, and understanding the essential handoffs that occur in a process. Exhibit 9.5 shows simple deployment flowcharts illustrating coordination between an orthodontist and oral surgeon in the care of the teenage patient described in Exhibit 7.1.

Using a flowchart to document a process allows managers and teams to see a picture of the process. Often just seeing a picture of the process leads to obvious ideas for improvement. Additional benefits include the opportunity to distinguish the distinct steps involved; identify unnecessary steps; understand vulnerabilities where breakdowns, mistakes, or delays are likely to occur; detect rework loops that contribute to inefficiency and quality waste; and define who carries out which step and when. The process of discussing, reviewing, and documenting a process using a flowchart provides the opportunity for clarifying operating assumptions (see double-loop learning

EXHIBIT 9.5
Simple
Deployment
Flowcharts

Vertical
Flowchart

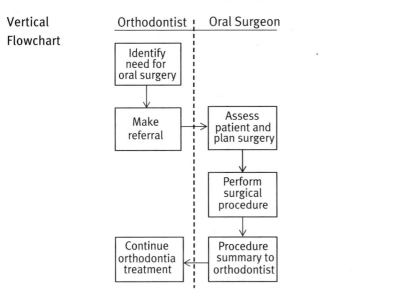

Horizontal Flowchart

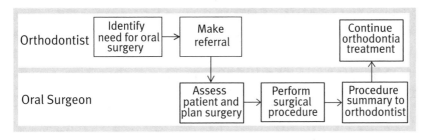

in Chapter 3), identifying variation in practice, and establishing agreement on how work should be done.

Prioritize the Problem

A **cause-and-effect diagram** is a tool for organizing and documenting causes of a problem in a structured format (Scholtes, Joiner, and Streibel 2003). The diagram may capture actual (observed) causes and/or possible (from brainstorming) causes. Because this diagram resembles a fish (the head represents the problem and the bones represent the causes), it is also referred to as a fishbone diagram (see Exhibit 9.6). The problem is written on the far right of the diagram. Categories of causes are represented by the diagonal lines (bones) connected to the horizontal line (spine), which leads to the problem (head). The bones of the fish may be labeled in a variety of ways to represent categories of causes, including people, plant and equipment, policies, procedures, manpower, methods, and materials.

Exhibit 9.7 is an example of a fishbone diagram. The problem is stated at the head of the fish (low hand-hygiene compliance) and the categories

Cause-and-effect diagram
(also referred to as a fishbone or Ishikawa diagram) a tool for organizing and documenting causes of a problem in a structured format

EXHIBIT 9.6

How the
Fishbone
Diagram Got
Its Name

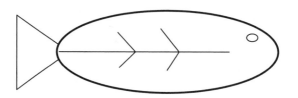

EXHIBIT 9.7

Fishbone
Diagram
Example

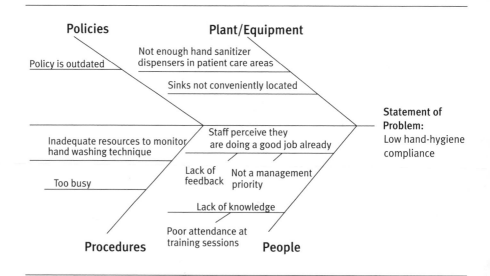

Pareto chart
bar graph that
displays data in
descending order
and also displays
cumulative totals
using a line graph
when reading
from left to right

Pareto Principle
"most effects
come from rela-
tively few causes;
that is, 80 percent
of the effects come
from 20 percent
of the possible
causes" (ASQ
2011, 54)

---

of causes are labeled as policies, procedure, people, and plant/equipment. Detailed causes are identified and represented by the small bones of the fish shown in the people category.

Stating the problem is the most important step in using the fishbone diagram. Problem statements that are too narrow, too vague, or poorly constructed can limit this tool's effectiveness in the improvement process. Users may be tempted to begin generating solutions (rather than document causes) in a fishbone diagram; however, users should take care to focus on causes because identifying solutions too soon also limits the tool's use and the opportunity to further investigate the problem.

Not all identified causes influence the problem equally. Data about how important causes are or how often causes occur aid managers in prioritizing and in turn selecting improvement interventions. A **Pareto chart** is a simple bar graph that displays data in descending order (most important/most frequent to least important/least frequent) and also displays cumulative totals using a line graph when reading from left to right. The Pareto chart is named after nineteenth-century economist Vilfredo Pareto and refers to the **Pareto Principle**, which suggests "most effects come from relatively

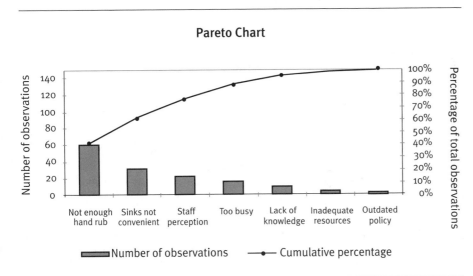

EXHIBIT 9.8
Pareto Chart
Example

few causes; that is, 80 percent of the effects come from 20 percent of the possible causes" (ASQ 2011, 54).

Exhibit 9.8 is an example of a Pareto chart based on data collected about the causes in Exhibit 9.7. Prior to collecting and displaying the data, the manager may have planned an educational session (e.g., how to wash hands). After systematically analyzing the problem, the manager realizes that the cause is the availability of supplies. He installs more hand sanitizer dispensers and provides small bottles for staff to carry in their pockets.

Improve the Process

Techniques such as Lean and Six Sigma (see Chapter 1), human factors engineering (Norman 2002; Gosbee 2005), and error proofing (Blanton et al. 2007) guide managers on how to improve a process once the underlying process problems are identified. These guidelines include: make it easy to do the right thing, minimize handoffs, find and remove bottlenecks, eliminate rework loops and unnecessary duplication, and use reminders.

Monitor Progress and Hold the Gains

A **run chart** is a graphic representation of data over time. Run charts track progress after an improvement intervention and monitor the performance of ongoing operations. On a run chart, the x-axis represents the time interval (e.g., day, month, quarter, or year) and the y-axis represents the **variable** or **attribute** of interest. Displaying data on a run chart also enables a manager to more readily detect patterns or unusual occurrences in the data. Exhibit 9.9 shows a run chart tracking hand-hygiene compliance. The intervention of installing more hand rub dispensers is indicated with the arrow.

Run chart
a graphic representation of data over time where the x-axis represents the time interval and the y-axis represents the variable of interest

Variables
also referred to as continuous data, "take on different values on a continuous scale" (Carey and Lloyd 2001, 70)

Attributes
also referred to as discrete data, "counts of events that can be aggregated into discrete categories" (Carey and Lloyd 2001, 70)

EXHIBIT 9.9

Run Chart of Hand-Hygiene Compliance by Percentage of Staff Observed Demonstrating Compliance

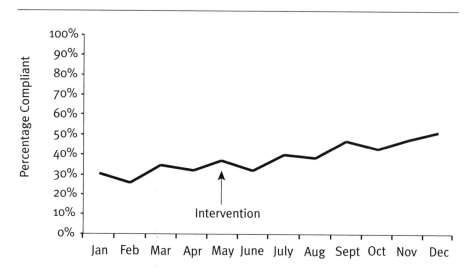

Root Cause Analysis

Serious problems may be investigated to better understand the causes and to identify actions to prevent their recurrence. The tool used to conduct this type of retrospective investigation is an in-depth root cause analysis (RCA). In the case of a sentinel event (see Chapter 7), The Joint Commission requires accredited organizations to conduct an RCA; develop and implement risk reduction strategies that target the identified root causes; and measure the effectiveness or results of the interventions (Joint Commission 2007). The Joint Commission defines an RCA as the following (Joint Commission 2007).

> A root cause analysis focuses primarily on systems and processes, not individual performance. It progresses from special causes in clinical processes to common causes in organizational processes and identifies potential improvements in processes or systems that would tend to decrease the likelihood of such events in the future, or determines, after analysis, that no such improvement opportunities exist.

Note: the terms "special cause" and "common cause" are discussed further in the next chapter.

This type of RCA is designed to aid organizations to systematically identify and better understand the patterns and systemic structures that contributed to the event. Several questions from The Joint Commission's RCA framework are shown in Exhibit 9.10. When the questions are grouped according to categories, the framework resembles the organizational levels illustrated in the iceberg metaphor (Exhibit 9.11).

Proximate Causes

- What human factors were relevant to the event?
- How could equipment performance affect the outcome?
- What controllable factors directly affected the outcome?
- Were there uncontrollable external factors?
- What other areas or services are impacted?

System and Process Underlying Causes

- To what degree is staff properly qualified and currently competent for their responsibilities?
- How did actual staffing compare with ideal levels?
- What are the plans for dealing with contingencies that would reduce effective staffing levels?
- How has staff performance in the relevant processes been assessed? When was this last performed?
- How can orientation and in-service training be improved?
- To what degree is necessary information available when needed?
- To what degree is communication among participants adequate?
- To what degree was the physical environment appropriate for the processes being carried out?
- What systems are in place to identify environmental risks?
- To what degree is the culture conducive to risk identification and reduction?
- What are the barriers to communication of potential risk factors?
- To what degree is the prevention of adverse outcomes communicated as a high priority?
- What can be done to protect against the effects of uncontrollable factors?

Source: From The Joint Commission. 2009. "A Framework for a Root Cause Analysis and Action Plan in Response to a Sentinel Event." Oakbrook Terrace, IL: The Joint Commission. Reprinted with permission.

EXHIBIT 9.10

The Joint Commission's Tool for Conducting a Root Cause Analysis: An Excerpt

Prospective Analysis

Problems may also be anticipated and processes improved in advance of a problem occurring. This proactive, preventive approach is referred to as a **prospective analysis**. **Failure mode and effects analysis (FMEA)** is a commonly used tool in prospective analysis.

Anyone who lost documents and wasted hours of work in the early days of personal computers can appreciate the periodic auto save, the pop-up warning of a low battery, and the rescued document features that are commonplace for users of contemporary computers. These features illustrate computer designers' understanding of the consequences of hardware and software failures on their users and the subsequent incorporation of product designs that prevent the failure from occurring (e.g., save the document before the battery runs out) or the user from incurring the consequences of the failure (e.g., document saved in the event of a sudden and unexpected power failure). Such is the premise of the FMEA.

Prospective analysis
a proactive, preventive approach to improvement that anticipates potential problems and improves processes in advance of a problem occurring

EXHIBIT 9.11

The Joint
Commission
Root Cause
Analysis

What happened? What are the details of the event?	Why did it happen? What were the most proximate factors?	Why did it happen? What systems and processes underlie those proximate factors?
• When • Where • What • Who	• The process or activity in which the event occurred • Human factors • Equipment factors • Controllable environmental factors	• Human resources issues • Information management issues • Environmental management issues • Leadership issues (corporate culture, encouragement of communication, clear communication of priorities) • Uncontrollable factors
Events	*Patterns*	*Systemic structures*

Source: Adapted from The Joint Commission. 2009. "A Framework for a Root Cause Analysis and Action Plan in Response to a Sentinel Event."

FMEA (failure mode and effects analysis)
a systematic process used to conduct a prospective analysis

Just as the continuous improvement cycle discussed earlier in the chapter represents systemic ways of thinking about improvement, FMEA represents a systemic way of thinking of patient safety and medical errors. "Systemic analysis . . . requires a simultaneous imagining of all possible stories . . . FMEA [does not] refer to a specific methodology; instead . . . [it] defines terms of inquiry . . . 'what has failed, what could fail, and how?'. . . . Given the various possibilities for failure, what are the potential consequences of each?' . . . [I]n general, a failure is said to occur if a component or a collection of components of a system behaves in a way that is not included in its specified performance criteria" (Senders and Senders 1999, 3.2–3.3).

This type of analysis has been used for many years by chemical, structural, mechanical, software, and aerospace engineers. Use of FMEA in healthcare is growing, particularly since The Joint Commission redesigned its accreditation standards. The standards initially required healthcare facilities to identify and conduct at least one FMEA on a high-risk process every year and have evolved to integrate management of risks throughout the standards (see Chapter 8). Common applications of the FMEA tool include medication and intravenous fluid administration, technology implementation, communication and handoffs, and product design. As with all of the tools described in this chapter, an FMEA is most effective when used in the context of a multidisciplinary team. Various forms, charts, and matrices to aid in conducting and documenting an FMEA may be found in the Web Resources box in this chapter.

Implementing Improvements

An understanding of systems provides implementation insights for managers. This section describes an implementation framework based on four system lessons: unintended consequences, "small wins," "begin with the end in mind," and creative tension.

Unintended Consequences

The principle of continuous improvement may be viewed as scalable; in other words, the size and scope of improvements may vary from very small to very large. While early efforts at improvement focused on continually improving an individual process, as presented in Chapter 6 an understanding of complex systems reveals that "we must almost always avoid focusing on just one element and pursuing only one goal; instead, we must pursue several goals at once" (Dorner 1996, 63–64). Managers must recognize that processes targeted for improvement interact with other processes within that system and are also "nested" within the larger system (Exhibit 9.12). When implementing improvements, managers must not only link improvements in a continuous manner to continually improve the system, but must also consider the effect of one improvement on the rest of the system.

In a large tertiary care hospital, one improvement effort was aimed at decreasing the amount of time patients spent on a ventilator after coronary bypass surgery. A patient's progress toward recovery could be greatly enhanced if less time was spent connected to a ventilator. The improvement team thoughtfully took into account the upstream influences on the patient recovery process by inviting operating room staff and an anesthesiologist to be members of the improvement team. However, no acute care patient-care representative was included.

After bypass surgery, when a patient met the required clinical criteria, she was transferred from the ICU to the acute care patient-care unit. After

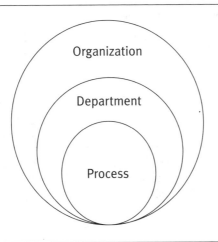

EXHIBIT 9.12
Nested Systems

the new ICU protocol was put into place, patients who had coronary bypass surgery began arriving in the acute care unit a day earlier and were sicker than patients who had been transferred under the old protocol. Although these patients were not on ventilators, the early transfer made a difference in other aspects of their care. The acute care unit found itself short staffed on numerous occasions. Although the same number of nurses was being scheduled, the higher patient acuity, which required more intense nursing care, led to the unit's understaffing.

After several weeks, the nurses in the acute care unit realized that a change had been made in the ICU's postoperative process. The nurse manager took several months to hire the required staff to meet the new acuity demands, during which time the existing nurses remained short staffed and overworked.

Anticipating, identifying, measuring, and proactively managing unintended consequences should be considered in any implementation plan. Exhibit 9.13 illustrates how this ICU improvement team might have identified unintended consequences by asking not only "Who/what affects our process?" but also "Who/what is affected by our process?" Asking this question early in the improvement effort would have allowed earlier coordination with those affected and reduced the negative impact of unintended consequences.

Another example of unintended consequences may be seen in how some institutions implement privacy policies. An elderly patient with an infection was admitted to the hospital in a confused state. Her daughter was denied information about her condition even though the daughter was her mother's designated medical proxy. Although the medical power of attorney documents were included in the patient's chart, the emergency department (ED) nurse refused to give out any information because the daughter was not on this patient's designated "approved visitor list" at the nurse's station. Because the well-intended privacy policies did not account for this particular circumstance, they actually interfered with communicating vital patient information to the ED care providers.

A lack of understanding and failure to anticipate unintended consequences may be considered a management planning error (see Chapter 4).

EXHIBIT 9.13

Anticipating Unintended Consequences

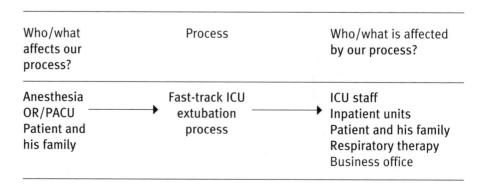

Who/what affects our process?	Process	Who/what is affected by our process?
Anesthesia OR/PACU Patient and his family	Fast-track ICU extubation process	ICU staff Inpatient units Patient and his family Respiratory therapy Business office

A lack of monitoring unintended consequences after implementing a change may be considered a management execution error (Reason 1995).

Small Wins

Using a small-wins strategy for implementing improvements within the larger system recognizes the dynamic complexity inherent in health services organizations (see Chapter 2). "Small wins provide information that facilitates learning and adaptation. Small wins are like miniature experiments that test implicit theories about resistance and opportunity and uncover both resources and barriers that were invisible before the situation was stirred up. . . . [A] series of small wins is also more structurally sound . . . because small wins are stable building blocks" (Weick 1984, 44).

Karl Weick, noted psychologist, defines a **small win** within the context of addressing social problems as (1984, 43)

> a concrete, complete, implemented outcome of moderate importance. By itself, one small win may seem unimportant. A series of wins at small but significant tasks, however, reveals a pattern that may attract allies, deter opponents, and lower resistance to subsequent proposals. Small wins are controllable opportunities that produce visible results.

> **Small win**
> "a concrete, complete, implemented outcome of moderate importance"
> (Weick 1984, 43)

This approach not only promotes continuous improvement but capitalizes on knowledge gained about system structure along the way. The benefits for managers are that small wins preserve gains and cannot unravel; they require less coordination to execute and they are minimally affected by leadership, management, or administrative changes or turnover (Weick 1984, 44). For employees, small wins are less stressful and are easier to comprehend and view as achievable. As a result, employees are more likely to comply with a small-wins intervention (Weick 1984, 44, 45).

Begin with the End in Mind

Consider two approaches to purchasing a new home. Every day for a week, Person A searches the real-estate advertisements in the newspapers. His diligent search yields some properties that he is interested in, so he calls a Realtor for a tour of each. After seeing a certain property, he immediately knows it is his perfect house. The Realtor refers him to a mortgage company to work out the financing. Person A is confident that no problem will arise because, based on his own calculations, his salary will cover the monthly payments. But then he receives the bad news: he does not qualify for the financing. Payments on a new car bought six months earlier, outstanding credit card bills from a recent vacation, and insufficient savings all work against him. Person A only qualifies for a loan that is too small for his dream home.

Person A's coworker, Person B, has a hobby of scanning the real-estate news. For years, Person B has been watching trends, and so she has identified a particular area of the city in which she would like to purchase a house. Based on the average housing prices in that area, Person B calculates what she will need for a down payment and for monthly mortgage payments. She systematically accumulates the funds for the down payment, makes sure she pays her credit card balances down to zero every month, and prequalifies with a mortgage company. Although most of her friends and coworkers drive new cars, her car is five years old but completely paid for. When Person B's "perfect house" comes on the market, she is the first to see it and is able to complete the purchase without a problem. When Person A overhears Person B talking about her new address, Person A cannot believe it; he wonders, "How could she possibly afford that place when she makes the same salary as I do?"

The answer to Person A's question is that these coworkers used two entirely different approaches to planning and implementing their processes for house buying. Person A used an approach called "forward planning," which involves taking one step at a time and not knowing the next step until after the previous step is completed. Person B used an approach called "reverse planning" (Dorner 1996), which involves defining the desired result—in this case, her ideal house—and then working backward to determine a practical or logical starting point to the step-by-step process of getting to the result. In reverse planning, each step is a necessary precondition to the next step. By planning in this manner, Person B could make purposeful choices (e.g., not buying a new car, reducing her credit card debt) that would help her toward, rather than become barriers to, the goal of purchasing her ideal house.

Similar approaches have been described in the literature. Habit number two in *The Seven Habits of Highly Effective People* by Stephen Covey (1990) advises to "begin with the end in mind." The "solution after next" principle, from *Breakthrough Thinking: The Seven Principles of Creative Problem Solving*, indicates that more effective solutions may be generated "by working backward from an ideal target solution for the future" (Nadler and Hibino 1994).

Creative Tension

The Animal Control Services team at a county health department recognized that the community had a huge problem. The past several years had seen an increase in county pet populations, stray animals, and animal bites. In addition, rabies had reemerged after the county had been rabies-free for years. The team made some progress when it instituted a 100-percent-sterilization requirement for adopted animals. Although the department offered pet sterilization to any animal currently being adopted, because the process was cumbersome, many owners did not follow up once they took their new pet home, and some decided against adopting altogether. The team had an idea to redesign the pet adoption process that would enable pets to be sterilized before they left the animal shelter rather than having the new owner assume the responsibility for sterilization.

The challenge was that the new plan would require some allocation of funds from the county commissioners. The team realized the importance of this public health issue; however, they were faced with the problem of how to communicate their sense of urgency to an audience with little knowledge of the issue. Faced with only five minutes on the county commissioner's agenda, the team decided on the following approach: present the facts and share the vision of a successful program. The veterinarian director of the team started the presentation with the following:

> Start with one female dog. . . . [I]n the first year, she produces an average of eight puppies, four of them females . . . in the second year, production of first and second generation females is 40 pups, 20 of them females . . . in the third year, production from three generations of females is 200 pups . . . in the fourth year, production from four generations is 1,000 . . . and so on. . . . [B]y the eighth generation, this one female pup has resulted in the production of 625,000 puppies!!! (McNeil et al. 2002)

After the veterinarian gave a few statistics on animal bites and rabies and a brief overview of the plan for the new pet adoption process, the county commissioners were sold. A local reporter concluded a column describing the Animal Control Services' proposal with this comment: "The only question at this point would seem to be, is it possible to move faster?" (*Wilmington Morning Star* 2002).

Animal Control Services understood how to use creative tension to engage stakeholders, gain support for its vision, and jump-start its improvement effort. First, it stated the facts, which in this case were the reproductive capacity of one female puppy and the health consequences of pet overpopulation. Next, it offered its vision of a process. Finally, by clearly revealing the performance gap between what currently existed and what was possible, the team used the concept of creative tension to establish the traction needed to get its effort moving forward (McNeil et al. 2002).

Just as the medical specialty of surgery consists of such subspecialties as neurosurgery, orthopedic surgery, and plastic surgery, the field of systems thinking also consists of subfields. One of these subfields is called "structural dynamics." Tension resolution is the fundamental building block in structural dynamics (Fritz 1996). When a difference exists between one thing and another, the resulting discrepancy creates the tendency toward movement. One type of tension found in organizations is called **creative tension**, which is formed by the discrepancy between an organization's current level of performance and its desired level and vision for the future.

Creative tension
the discrepancy between an organization's current level of performance and its desired level and vision for the future

The rubber-band metaphor has been used to illustrate the concept of creative tension (Senge 1990). Think of holding a rubber band, with one end in each hand and one hand above the other. Stretch the rubber band, and feel the tension of the pull. Think of the higher hand as vision—that is, the desired future state of the organization. Think of the lower hand as current reality—that is, the current level of the organization's performance. The tension may be released from the rubber band by only three ways.

The first way to relieve tension is to let go of the end clasped by the lower hand. As the tension is released, the rubber band is drawn to the top hand. The greater the tension, the faster and more strongly the rubber band will return to the top hand. In organizations, this tension resolution may be seen as drawing the organization toward a vision. The second way to relieve tension is to let go of the end clasped by the higher hand. As the tension is released, the rubber band is drawn to the bottom hand. In organizations, this tension resolution may be seen as maintaining the status quo or stagnating. The third way to relieve tension is by stretching the rubber band beyond its natural limit and breaking it. In organizations, this type of tension resolution may be seen in situations where too much is expected, too fast, and without adequate resources; as a result, people and processes "break." Symptoms of this last type of tension resolution include employee turnover, morale problems, poor performance, and medical errors.

When organizational change and performance are viewed through a systems perspective, tension resolution is the key tool for changing behavior. The essential elements for creative tension to be present in an organization are current reality, vision, and an actual or perceived gap between the two. The manager's role is to consciously generate, make visible, and regulate creative tension in the organization to leverage the resulting tendency toward movement (Heifetz and Laurie 2001). Adopting the philosophy of continuous standards compliance (Chapter 8) and using the performance management cycle (Exhibit 9.3) aid managers in this work.

SWOT
strengths, weaknesses, opportunities, threats analysis

PEST
political, economic, social, technological analysis

The first requirement for creative tension, vision, is discussed in Chapter 5. The second requirement for creative tension is a common, objective description of current reality. Performance measurement (Chapter 10) is one way managers describe current reality; organizational assessment is another. Organizational assessment and diagnosis may be more familiar to strategic planners who have used **SWOT** (strengths, weaknesses, opportunities, threats) or **PEST** (political, economic, social, technological) analyses or to organizational development professionals than to managers. However, assessment offers a valuable way for managers to document, communicate, and promote a shared understanding of current reality. An organizational assessment or self-assessment simply refers to a systematic or repeatable method of examining the organization for its strengths and performance gaps. The Baldrige Performance Excellence Program Health Care Criteria for Performance Excellence systems model (see Chapter 4) is an important guide for organizational self-assessment. An organizational self-assessment conducted at regular intervals (e.g., annually, biannually) provides managers with the opportunity and impetus to systematically reexamine, document, and communicate current reality relative to desired organizational activities, strategies, and performance results.

Without a clear picture of current reality those within the organization will define reality on the basis of their own mental models, knowledge, and previous experiences. As a result, some may hold an overly positive view of the organization's current reality, and others may hold a disproportionately negative view. The net effect is the absence of a shared understanding of current reality and no shared understanding of the performance gap, which is necessary for creative tension. Creative tension creates tension resolution and, in turn, traction for change.

Framework for Implementation

A challenge for healthcare managers is that breakthrough technologies are most often associated with clinical breakthroughs in diagnosis (e.g., magnetic resonance imaging), intervention (e.g., minimally invasive surgery techniques), treatment (e.g., new drugs), or prevention (e.g., polio vaccination). Although specific technology breakthroughs are available that may enhance performance in the management domain (e.g., electronic information systems), management breakthroughs that influence organizational performance are most often associated with the environment in which the clinical technologies may be used. Management breakthroughs may be seen in (1) areas such as philosophies, approaches, and tools that enable managers to promote innovations in the operating environment, and (2) work processes that enable patients to fully realize the benefit of advancements in clinical technology.

Rather than the breakthrough resulting from a technical invention, the managerial breakthrough may be defined through the vision or context of the department, service, or organization. The ideal vision may stretch as far as needed to illuminate the performance gap and thus establish creative tension. Understanding the history of the organization, department, service, or technology helps managers identify and uncover issues, attitudes, or past events that may undermine implementation. An understanding of the past also promotes buy-in to change by grounding the change efforts by establishing continuity with past events (see Chapter 3). A clear statement of mission describes the purpose and justifies the existence of an organization, department, service, or process (Chapter 5). Implementing small wins in the direction of the vision represents continuous improvement within the system as it is defined. Exhibit 9.14 illustrates this conceptual framework for implementation, referred to as *breakthrough vision, incremental implementation* based on the previously described principles.

EXHIBIT 9.14

Implementation Framework: Breakthrough Vision, Incremental Implementation

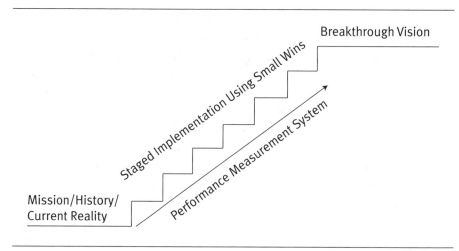

The steps taken toward achieving the vision must not be so great that they distract the care providers' focus and attention and place patient safety and outcomes at risk (Reason 1990). However, the steps taken in implementation must be large enough so that slipping back to the previous way of doing things is not possible. A step may have one or several concurrent interventions. Some interventions may be completed quickly, and others may be broken down and achieved in several sequential steps. The diagonal line beneath the steps that points toward the ideal vision is labeled "Performance Measurement System," indicating that progress toward the vision and measures of unintended consequences are continually monitored and evaluated.

Summary

Just as providers use the scientific method to systematically solve problems in the clinical arena, managers also should use systematic critical thinking approaches when designing improvements. Approaches introduced in this chapter include the PDCA cycle, the Six Sigma DMAIC cycle, and the performance improvement cycle. Numerous improvement tools to document and understand processes, to organize and analyze contributing causes to process problems, to prioritize problems, and to monitor improvements are available to managers. The breakthrough vision, incremental implementation framework takes into account lessons from complex systems. The approaches, tools, and framework discussed in this chapter can strengthen managers' ability to design and implement successful improvements while decreasing the likelihood of managerial planning and execution errors.

Exercise 1

Objective: To practice addressing the questions in The Joint Commission RCA tool.

Instructions:
- Read the following case scenario.
- Follow the instructions at the end of the case.

Case Study:
The letter in this case study is adapted with permission from Trina Bingham (2005), master's in nursing student at Duke University School of Nursing.

You are the risk manager of a tertiary care hospital and have just received the following letter from a patient who was recently discharged from your facility.

Dear Risk Manager,

Last month, I had surgery at your hospital. I was supposed to have a short laparoscopic surgery with a discharge by lunch, but it turned into an open surgery with complications. This led to a 4-day hospital stay and discharge with a Foley catheter. Overall, my hospital stay was OK, but I had a situation when the call bell was broken. It was during the night, and I was alone. I needed pain meds. I kept ringing the call bell and no one answered. I used my phone to call the switchboard and no one answered. I didn't want to yell. My IV began beeping (to be honest I kinked the tubing to make it beep), but no one came with that noise either. Eventually the certified nursing assistant (CNA) came to routinely check my vitals and she got a nurse for me. They switched call bells, but apparently there was an electrical problem, and the call bell couldn't be fixed until the next day when maintenance was working. The CNA told me to "holler if I needed anything" as she walked out closing the door. I was so mad, but by this time, the IV pain med was working and I was dozing off. I reported the situation again on day shift and spoke to the director of nursing and the quality assurance manager. Upon discharge, I included this dangerous and unethical situation on my patient satisfaction survey. But I have to wonder, when these data are combined with all the other data, if the situation looks insignificant. For me, it worked out OK. All I needed was pain medicine, but what if I had needed help for something more serious? Depending on the layout of satisfaction and quality of care survey results, this situation could look very minor. For all I know, my dissatisfaction was under the heading "dissatisfied with room."

I am writing to you because I have not heard from the director of nursing or the quality assurance manager about what they have done to fix the problems. I believe it is important that you hear my complaint so hopefully other patients will not have to go through the terrible experience that I did.

To fix the problems described in this patient's letter, you realize you must first understand the root causes of the problems. Although this situation did not result in a sentinel event, you realize that it could have and decide to conduct an RCA.

Brainstorm possible responses to the RCA questions in Exhibit 9.10.

Exercise 2

Objective: To gain an appreciation for a regular assessment of current reality in an organization.

Instructions:

- An integral activity in any healthcare provider–patient encounter involves the physical examination, checkup, or assessment. This exercise will examine what may be learned about the organizational examination, checkup, or assessment from this routine clinical practice.
- For questions *a* through *e*, you may choose to record your responses on the Assessment Worksheet following or on one similar to it.

  a. Describe the purpose of an annual physical examination. You may answer from a provider or patient point of view. You may discuss a physical examination, a well-child checkup, or a dental appointment.

  b. Describe the general sequence of events that occur during this examination.

  c. How do you (if you answered as a provider) or the provider (if you answered as a patient) know what to do to complete the examination?

  d. Describe why the examination is done in this particular way.

  e. Answer the same questions for an organization, and fill in the "Organizational Checkup" column in the worksheet.

Assessment Worksheet

	Physical Checkup	*Organizational Checkup*
Purpose		
Sequence of events		
How do you know what to do?		
Why is it done this way?		

f. On the basis of your responses to the previous questions, describe why managers should or should not perform organizational checkups on a routine basis.

Exercise 3

Objective: To practice anticipating unintended consequences.

Instructions:

- For questions *a* through *e*, you may choose to record your responses on the Unintended Consequences Worksheet following or on one similar to it.

    a. Select any process that takes place within a health services organization. Write that process in the center column, column A.

    b. Identify who (person, group, department, stakeholder) influences the process in column B. In other words, think about the activities and people upstream from your process.

    c. Identify who is influenced by the process in column C. In other words, think about the activities and people downstream from your process.

    d. Extend your response one more time. Identify who influences the items in column B. Write your response in column D.

    e. Identify who is influenced by the items in column C. Write your response in column E.

Unintended Consequences Worksheet

D	B	A	C	E
Who influences items in Column B	Who influences the process	The process	Who is influenced by the process	Who is influenced by items in Column C

   f. Describe one or two unintended consequences to a change in the process identified in column A.

Companion Readings

Anderson, J., L. L. Gosbee, M. Bessesen, and L. Williams. 2010. "Using Human Factors Engineering to Improve the Effectiveness of Infection Prevention and Control." *Critical Care Medicine* 38 (8 Suppl): S269–81.

Coles G., B. Fuller, K. Nordquist. S. Weissenberger, L. Anderson, and B. DuBois. 2010. "Three Kinds of Proactive Risk Assessments for Health Care." *The Joint Commission Journal on Quality and Patient Safety* 36 (8): 365–75.

Grosfeld, J. L. 2010. "Progress and Its Unintended Consequences." *American Journal of Surgery* 199 (3): 284–88.

Web Resources

Improvement Tools

American Society for Quality: www.asq.org/learn-about-quality/quality-tools
.html

Institute for Healthcare Improvement:
www.ihi.org/IHI/Topics/Improvement/ImprovementMethods/Tools

Embracing Quality in Local Public Health: Michigan's Quality Improvement
Guidebook: http://accreditation.localhealth.net/MLC-2%20website/
Michigans_QI_Guidebook.pdf

National Association of County and City Health Officials (NACCHO) Quality
Improvement Toolkit: www.naccho.org/toolbox/program
.cfm?id=25&display_name=Quality%20Improvement%20Toolkit

Patient Safety and Quality: An Evidence-Based Handbook for Nurses. AHRQ
Publication No. 08-0043. Chapter 44: "Tools and Strategies for
Quality Improvement and Patient Safety." www.ahrq.gov/qual/
nurseshdbk/docs/HughesR_QMBMP.pdf

Patient Safety

Institute for Safe Medication Practices: www.ismp.org

Veteran's Administration National Center for Patient Safety:
www.patientsafety.gov/index.html

Advances in Patient Safety: From Research to Implementation, Volumes 1–4:
www.ahrq.gov/qual/advances

Patient Safety Tools: Failure Mode and Effects Analysis/Root Cause Analysis

Veteran's Administration National Center for Patient Safety:
www.patientsafety.gov/SafetyTopics.html

Veteran's Administration National Center for Patient Safety:
www.patientsafety.gov/rca.html

The Joint Commission Sentinel Event Forms and Tools:
www.jointcommission.org/SentinelEvents/Forms/

Additional Resources

The Critical Thinking Community: www.criticalthinking.org

Scholtes, P. R., B. L. Joiner, and B. J. Streibel. 2003. *The Team Handbook,*
3rd ed. Madison, WI: Oriel Inc.

Ransom, E. R., M. S. Joshi, D. B. Nash, and S. B. Ransom (eds.). 2008. *The
Healthcare Quality Book: Vision, Strategy and Tools,* 2nd ed. Chicago:
Health Administration Press.

10

MEASURING PROCESS AND SYSTEM PERFORMANCE

Learning Objectives

After completing this chapter you should be able to:

- describe ways that a systems perspective influences how managers measure, analyze, manage, and improve performance;
- graphically analyze data to identify patterns and system structures;
- explore mental models associated with performance measurement;
- explain how performance measurement fits within the quality continuum; and
- identify sources of comparative performance data for health services organizations.

Every day we use data to make decisions and monitor our personal interests, whether we are following the progress of our favorite sports team (reviewing team rankings), determining how to dress (checking the weather report), shopping (calculating balance on a debit or credit card), or knowing when to mow the lawn (seeing the grass is too high).

People use data to guide their own healthcare activities, too. A child's hot forehead alerts a mother to the possibility of a fever. A grandfather with diabetes measures his daily blood glucose level to regulate his insulin dosage. People exercise 20 minutes a day, three times a week, to remain fit. Care providers use data to diagnose, treat, and monitor clinical conditions and the effectiveness of interventions. Blood tests, x-rays, and vital signs all provide information to enhance the care provider's effectiveness. In each of these examples, data add value to the process. Data give us information about something we are interested in, help us choose among various options, alert us when something needs to be done, and define the boundaries of an activity.

When we follow our favorite sports team during the course of the season, we are looking at data over time for trends and progress. When we check to see what place the team is in relation to the other teams in the same division, we are comparing data points. When we realize the grass is high compared with the neighbors', we are using a benchmark to signal that we need to mow it. If we check the weather report for the barometric pressure or chance of rain, we are using formal measures. When we use our hand to check a forehead for fever, we are measuring informally.

These measurement lessons from other parts of life are easily overlooked in the workplace. While immersed in data and reporting, health services managers face the risk of being "data rich and information poor" about how their unit, department, or organization is actually performing.

Traditional linear approaches to measuring and analyzing performance have limitations when applied to complex systems. This chapter provides measurement lessons to help managers better understand and improve system behavior.

Preserve the Context

Context
"the interrelated conditions in which something exists or occurs" (Merriam-Webster Dictionary Online 2010a)

Organizational context is described in Chapter 5. In regard to measurement, the term **context** refers to "the interrelated conditions in which something exists or occurs" (Merriam-Webster Dictionary Online 2010a). To illustrate, consider the three numbers 656, 1087, and 1049. What do the numbers mean? Say these three numbers are each associated with a month of the year: January = 656; March =1087; and June =1049. What do the numbers mean now? Add the descriptor: number of visits to an outpatient mammography center. What do the numbers mean now? This is the question faced by the mammography center manager. For several months the center's staff had been complaining about being busy. The manager needed to determine if the increase in visits was a permanent change or if it was a passing phenomenon. The monthly reports he received from the finance department presented the center's volume statistics in a spreadsheet according to this month, last month, year to date, and the same month, previous year. He used those reports to generate a run chart and was then able to determine the answer to his question (see Exhibit 10.1).

A "once every hundred years" snowstorm had hit the city the previous January and shut down business for four days. The center's current busy-ness was a reflection of the need to reschedule appointments that were cancelled as a result of the snowstorm. The overall volumes for the year were still on track; the monthly distribution of visits had been affected by this unusual and explainable event.

Consider another example. In this case, the internal medicine clinic of a large multispecialty physician practice implemented changes in its workflow to reduce patient waiting times and improve patient satisfaction. The improvements were implemented in September and at that time the satisfaction scores were 90 percent; in October, the satisfaction scores were 83 percent. Did the effort succeed or fail? Placing the satisfaction data in a run chart over time provides the context within which the September results should be interpreted (Exhibit 10.2).

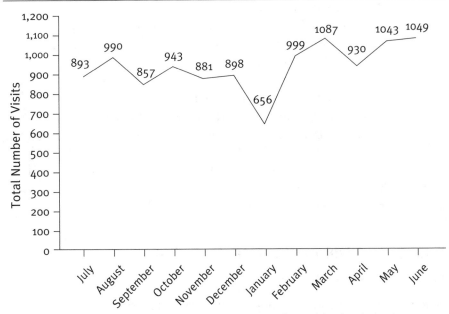

EXHIBIT 10.1

Breast Imaging Services Monthly Outpatient Visits

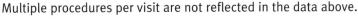

Multiple procedures per visit are not reflected in the data above.

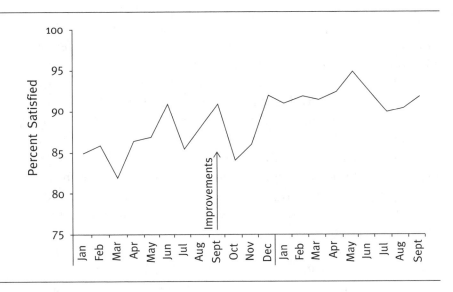

EXHIBIT 10.2

Patient Satisfaction Results

The run chart shows that patient satisfaction decreased the first month after the changes were implemented in September. This decline is not uncommon because new processes often take time to stabilize as a result of staff learning curves and adjustments. Managers must not overreact to one month's worth of data but should continue to track results over time to see the pattern of performance once the process has stabilized. This run chart demonstrates that although patient satisfaction dropped initially, in subsequent months it stabilized at a higher average level and that more consistent performance became apparent from month to month.

These two examples illustrate several principles about data and complex systems (Wheeler 2000, 14, 79):

- No data have meaning apart from their context.
- Graphs reveal interesting structures present in the data.
- Graphs make data more accessible to the human mind than do tables.

Identifying patterns in lists or tables of numbers is difficult. Run charts and other types of graphs enable managers to better see patterns, which in turn can provide clues to system structures.

Bundle and Unbundle Data According to the User's Purpose

When different levels of the organization are telling different stories about the operating environment, unbundling or disaggregating the indicators can be useful. For example, administrators of a large tertiary care hospital tracked staff turnover rates as one of the hospital's performance indicators. Turnover for the nursing department was 25 percent, which the administrators considered to be reasonable given the local employment and economic environments. However, the nurse managers and nurses consistently voiced their concerns about understaffing and turnover.

The aggregate turnover figures reflected the combined turnover of registered nurses, licensed practical nurses, certified nurse assistants, and unit secretaries. Unbundling the data revealed that although the departmental turnover was 25 percent, the registered nurse turnover was 15 percent and the certified nurse assistant turnover was 43 percent. While studying the departmental turnover data, the human resources department realized that internal staff transfers were not included in the turnover calculations; only terminations were included. When staff movement within the organization was also taken into account, it became apparent that the original turnover figures significantly underestimated the impact of staff changes on the nurse managers and the frontline nursing staffs. Once these flaws in the performance indicators were identified, the human resources department redesigned its performance indicators and reporting mechanisms to account for changing activity at the unit level in addition to aggregate turnover at the departmental or organizational level.

The "distinction between data and information does not lie in the content of a given string of characters. It lies more in its relationship to required decisions. [Data are] measurements that enable us to judge the impact of a local decision on the company's goal" (Goldratt 1990, 4, 10). In the previous example, although the hospital administrators were receiving data, originally they were not receiving information to best understand the relationship between their decisions and the organization's goals.

The selection and presentation of metrics should match the level and purpose of its user. Consider the following four levels of decision making in a hospital: board level, senior executive level, nursing service line level, and nursing unit level. Now consider the following examples of HCAHPS reports. The survey instrument contains the following questions (AHRQ 2011):

- During this hospital stay, how often did nurses treat you with courtesy and respect?
- During this hospital stay, how often did nurses listen carefully to you?
- During this hospital stay, how often did nurses explain things in a way you could understand?

The CMS Hospital Compare website combines the questions into one value (CMS 2011a): patients who reported that their nurses "always" communicated well. The summary indicator is presented monthly to the board and is shown in Exhibit 10.3. A summary report including the hospital-wide results for each question is generated for the senior executives and shown in Exhibit 10.4. Four inpatient units, reporting to one director, make up the medical-surgical inpatient nursing service line. A report containing the results for each question for all four units is generated for the nursing director. An example of one question is shown in Exhibit 10.5. Finally, a unit-based report with results for each question is generated for each unit manager. An example of results for three questions for one unit is shown in Exhibit 10.6.

The senior executive for quality and safety, responsible for designing and distributing the reports, understood the different data needs for the different decision makers. He also understood that as data are aggregated, some performance information may become buried in the data and that important opportunities for improvement may be missed. In this case, the director-level report provided key information for system improvement. Presented like this, the data revealed erratic performance on each of the four units. However, when one department is up, another is down, so when aggregated—as in the board-level and senior executive–level reports—the extremes canceled each other out. This key insight would be missed and leaders would be under the misimpression that patient perceptions were pretty consistent if the board-level or senior executive–level reports were the only ones reviewed in this organization. Overlaying multiple question results for Unit 4 on one graph demonstrates erratic performance on each question, indicating fundamental process problems with how care is organized and delivered and a lack of consistency among caregivers.

Because the senior executive for quality and safety also understood the importance of communicating the data's context, a brief explanation

EXHIBIT 10.3

Board-Level
Report: Nurse
Communi-
cation

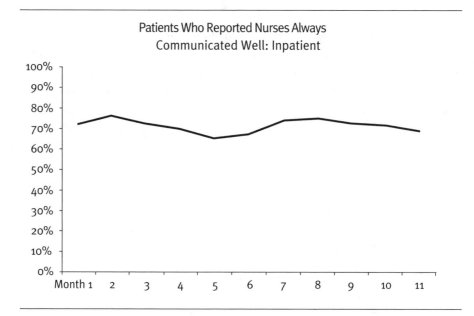

Patients Who Reported Nurses Always
Communicated Well: Inpatient

EXHIBIT 10.4

Senior
Executive–Level
Report: Nurse
Communication
by Question

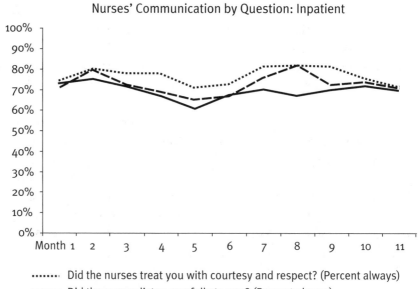

Nurses' Communication by Question: Inpatient

······· Did the nurses treat you with courtesy and respect? (Percent always)

--- Did the nurses listen carefully to you? (Percent always)

—— Did the nurses explain things in a way that you could understand?
(Percent always)

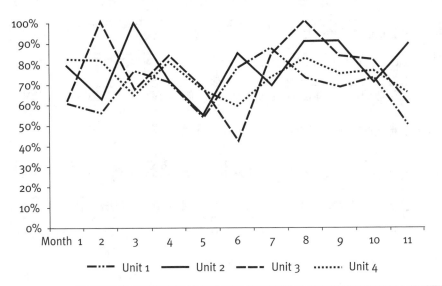

EXHIBIT 10.5
Service Line–
Level Report:
Individual
Question
Results by Unit
in the Service
Line

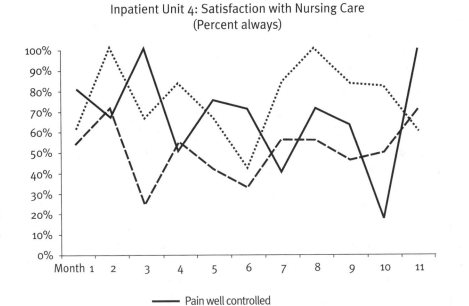

EXHIBIT 10.6
Unit Manager–
Level Report:
Individual
Question
Results for
Unit 4 Only

EXHIBIT 10.7

Sample Hospital Financial Scorecard

	Hospital XYZ Year 1	Year 2	Bench mark facility	Regional Median	U.S. Median	Rating[1]	Rating Dashboard (see key)	Trend (see key)
Financial Overview								
Total Margin	0.40	(3.00)	2.00	2.07	3.70	Fair	★ ★	⇧
Market Factors								
Inpatient Revenue %	60.6	65.1	63.9	62.3	55.5	Fair	★ ★	ⱴ
Investment Efficiency								
Days in A/R	54	55	80	56	56	Average	★ ★ ★	
Plant Obsolescence								
Average Age of Plant	17.0	N/A	8.2	N/A	9.6	Poor	★	
Capital Position								
Debt Financing %	104.0	104.8	48.7	57.7	47.8	Poor	★	
Labor Costs								
Staffing								
FTEs per Adjusted Patient Day	4.7	4.9	7.2	4.9	4.7	Average	★ ★ ★	⇩
Supply Costs								
Avg. Medical Supply Cost per Medicare Discharge (CMI = 1.0)	602	449	1,454	778	660	Average	★ ★ ★	⬆
Non-Operating Income								
Days Cash on Hand	17	14	29	55	36	Fair	★ ★	⇧

Key:

Favorable trend, measure is increasing ⇧   Favorable trend, measure is decreasing ⇩
Unfavorable trend, measure is increasing ⬆ Unfavorable trend, measure is decreasing ⬇
The measure has increased by > 2%, but the change must be interpreted with respect to additional measures ⋏
The measure has decreased by > 2%, but the change must be interpreted with respect to additional measures ⱴ
Rating Scale: poor, fair, average, good, and excellent, represented by 1–5 stars, respectively. Ratings are based on comparisons with national data.

Notes:

The far right column of the pages with the individual performance measures provides trend information, when available. This trend information should be interpreted cautiously. An arrow in this column is simply a mathematical indicator. It tells only whether this performance measure changed by more than two percent compared with the prior year. As such, there is no inherent judgment value contained in this information. *The purpose is simply to highlight measures that are changing so that, if appropriate, they can be studied further.* Even an unfavorable trend might not really be bad news. For example, suppose that some cost measure increased by 3%, which would be flagged as an unfavorable trend. If local, regional, and US hospitals experienced a 6% increase in this measure, this increase could be considered quite good relative to what was experienced elsewhere and probably reflects excellent managerial performance. *Furthermore, executives generally would want to avoid extreme values of any measure* (italics added).

Source: Reprinted with permission from Andrew Cameron, PhD, MBA. Principal, Mantium Consulting Services.

accompanied each report as data were aggregated; the director and unit manager–level reports included all four levels of data so they could see how their performance fit within the performance of the organization overall.

Many health services organizations have adopted a "report card" or "scorecard" approach to present a quick visual summary of the organization's current performance status to senior executives and the board. Analysis is conveyed through red-yellow-green schematics or arrows going up, down, or horizontal. However, the desire for brevity sometimes leads to a loss of context. Exhibit 10.7 is an excerpt from a sample financial scorecard that maintains the balance between brevity and context. Noteworthy are the key and notes guiding readers to the context within which the ratings and trends should be interpreted.

These examples illustrate two principles about data and complex systems (Wheeler 2000, 105):

1. As data are aggregated they lose their context and usefulness.
2. Aggregated data may be used as a report card, but they will not pin-point what needs to be fixed.

Chapter 8 uses the iceberg metaphor to illustrate that an understanding of systemic structure (below the waterline) helps managers target system changes that guide process improvements, which in turn improve care to the individual patient (events). In other words, the direction of managerial actions follows the arrows shown in Exhibit 8.9. Similarly, aggregated data may be considered "above the waterline"; unbundling, sorting, and retaining the context of the data help managers go below the waterline to understand what needs to be improved.

Differentiate Types of Measures and Their Uses

To understand, use, and communicate quality metrics, managers must be able to differentiate between types of metrics and their respective characteristics. Exhibit 10.8 clarifies assumptions associated with different types of quality measurements: those used for research, improvement, and accountability.

These three types of measures provide valuable above-the-waterline information when choosing interventions and implementing improvements, and for determining the degree to which one compares to a defined standard. However, on their own, these measures provide limited information for the manager to better understand system behavior.

To address managerial needs for quality performance metrics, the category "performance management measures" must be added to Exhibit 10.8. In Chapter 9, the performance management cycle was introduced as a continuous improvement model for the managerial domain. The business literature defines **performance management** as "an umbrella term that describes the methodologies, metrics, processes and systems used to monitor and manage the business performance of an enterprise" (Buytendijk and Rayner 2002). Performance management is also referred to as *enterprise performance management* (EPM), *corporate performance management* (CPM), and *business performance management* (BPM).

The difference between performance management measures and research measures may be compared to the difference between descriptive and analytic epidemiological studies.

> Descriptive studies are concerned with characterizing the amount and distribution of disease within a population. Analytic studies, on the other hand, are concerned with the determinants of disease, the reasons for relatively high or low frequency of disease in specific population subgroups. Descriptive studies usually precede analytic studies: the former are used to identify any health problems that

Performance management "an umbrella term that describes the methodologies, metrics, processes and systems used to monitor and manage the business performance of an enterprise" (Buytendijk and Rayner 2002)

EXHIBIT 10.8
Key Aspects of
Performance
Measurement
by Type

Aspect	Research	Improvement	Accountability
Measurement aim	New knowledge	Improvement of care	Comparison [with standards, benchmarks, other organizations (Baars 2009)], choice, reassurance, spur for change
Measurement methods (test observability)	Test blinded or controlled	Test observable	No test, evaluate current performance
Bias	Designed to eliminate bias	Accept consistent bias	Measure and adjust to reduce bias
Sample size	"Just in case" data	"Just enough" data, small sequential samples	Obtain 100% of available, relevant data
Flexibility of hypothesis	Fixed hypothesis	Hypothesis is flexible; it changes as learning takes place	No hypothesis
Testing strategy	One large test	Sequential tests	No tests
Determining if change is an improvement	Hypothesis, statistical test (t-test, F-test, chi-square) with p-values	Run charts of Shewhart control charts (use statistical process control methods)	No change focus
Confidentiality of data	Research subjects' identities protected	Data used only by those involved with improvement	Data available for public consumption and review

Source: Adapted and reprinted with permission from Lloyd, R. 2010. "Helping Leaders Blink Correctly." *Healthcare Executive* 25 (3): 88–91.

may exist, and the latter proceed to identify the cause(s) of the problem. (Friis and Sellers 2009, 143)

Descriptive studies provide the foundation for public health surveillance, defined as "the systematic process of identifying, collecting, orderly summarization, analysis, and evaluation of data . . . with the prompt dissemination of findings to those who need to know and need to take action" (Oleske 2009, 138). Friis and Sellers (2009) define the purpose of descriptive epidemiological data to evaluate trends and identify emerging problems, inform planning, and identify areas for further study by analytic methods. Performance management measures may be thought of as the organizational surveillance system to monitor ongoing performance, or the descriptive data that provide clues about the determinants of system behavior (i.e., below-the-waterline structures) and offer direction for further investigation. Performance management measures may be used to generate hypotheses, but are not used to test hypotheses or define the strength of relationships or causation.

The difference between performance management measures and improvement measures may be compared to the difference between epidemiology methods and improvement methods. Improvement methods are used when a defined process is not performing as well as desired or if a solution is available but is difficult to implement. Epidemiological methods are used when outcomes are present but the underlying processes (i.e., determinants) generating the outcomes are not known (Kritchevsky and Simmons 1995). Similarly, improvement measures, using run charts, help identify patterns or trends within a process or groups of related processes. Performance management measures help identify patterns across processes to better understand the underlying system causes or structures generating the system outcomes.

The difference between performance management measures and accountability measures is seen in their fundamental purpose. The purpose of accountability measures is comparison to a given standard; in other words, evaluation. Within the context of systems thinking and improving system performance, the purpose of performance management measures is to provide feedback about the system's behavior—in other words, understanding. Feedback about the system's behavior provides clues about systemic structure. Understanding systemic structure enables one to manage from below the waterline (see Chapter 3).

The characteristics of performance management measures may be described according to the same elements as research, improvement, and accountability measures. These characteristics are summarized in Exhibit 10.9 according to the elements mentioned previously.

Select a Balanced Set of Measures

As discussed in Chapter 7, customer, stakeholder, and market requirements are the foundation for and drive all work performed by the organization. Not only do these requirements guide process design but they also define criteria against which process and organizational effectiveness are determined.

Organizations must purposefully select performance indicators that are linked to and aligned with their organizations' goals, business strategy, and customer and stakeholder requirements. Integrating internal and external measurement requirements may also be thought of in terms of a Venn diagram. In Exhibit 10.10, one circle represents internally driven performance

EXHIBIT 10.9

Performance
Management
Measures

Aspect	Performance Management
Measurement aim	Feedback about system performance
Measurement methods (Test Observability)	Descriptive
Bias	Measure and adjust to reduce bias and/or accept consistent bias
Sample size	Obtain 100% of available, relevant data
Flexibility of hypothesis	Used to generate hypotheses
Testing strategy	No tests; observe for trends, patterns, variation
Determining if change is an improvement	Identify random and assignable variation
Confidentiality of data	Data presentation aligned with user's purpose; free information flow within the system

*Balanced
scorecard (BSC)*
A "set of measures
that gives top
managers a fast
but comprehen-
sive view of the
business. The bal-
anced scorecard
includes financial
measures and it
complements the
financial measures
with operational
measures on cus-
tomer satisfaction,
internal processes,
and the organiza-
tion's innovation
and improvement
activities—opera-
tional measures
that are the drivers
of future financial
performance."
(Kaplan and Nor-
ton 2005, 174)

measures, while the other circle represents externally driven performance measures. To leverage time, effort, and resources, managers should strategically select measures that allow for the largest area of overlap between the circles. In this way, performance measures may be used for multiple purposes internally and externally.

One approach to selecting measures is the **balanced scorecard** (BSC), a

set of measures that gives top managers a fast but comprehensive view of the business. The balanced scorecard includes financial measures that tell the results of actions already taken. And it complements the financial measures with operational measures on customer satisfaction, internal processes, and the organization's innovation and improvement activities—operational measures that are the drivers of future financial performance. (Kaplan and Norton 2005, 174)

Since its introduction 20 years ago, the BSC has progressed from a framework of performance metrics to a strategic management system (Kaplan and Norton 2007) and its use in healthcare organizations continues to grow and evolve (Gurd and Gao 2008). Exhibit 10.11 illustrates a simple balanced scorecard for an obstetrics practice. These department-specific measures are aligned with the organization's overall strategy of improving the customer's experience while delivering safe, quality, cost-effective services.

The clinical value compass may be thought of as a balanced scorecard for evaluating outcomes of a clinical process. The four categories that it measures (the points of the compass) are functional status and well-being, satisfaction against need, costs, and clinical status (Nelson et al. 1996). These four points may be used to measure, evaluate, and improve the effectiveness

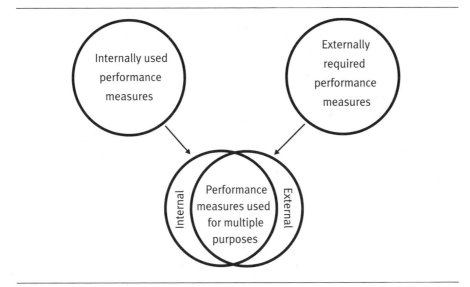

EXHIBIT 10.10
Leveraging
Performance
Measures

Customer
- Patient and family satisfaction
- Market share
- Referral rates

Innovation and Learning
- Staff credentials and certifications
- Hours of inservice education
- Improvement teams per year

Internal
- C-section rates
- Maternal complications
- Neonatal complications
- Monitoring capacity

Financial
- Cost per delivery
- Nurse-to-patient ratio
- Supply costs
- Turnover rates

EXHIBIT 10.11
Simple
Obstetrics
Balanced
Scorecard

of a clinical process, and they may also serve as a guide for managers when selecting metrics to measure, evaluate, and improve the performance of their departments or organizations.

Performance management measures may also be grouped according to Donabedian's (1980) three types of medical quality indicators: structure measures, process measures, and outcome measures. Tools, resources, characteristics of providers, settings, and organizations are considered structure measures; examples of these types of measures are the number of hospital beds, the number of physicians on staff, and the age of the radiology equipment. Activities that occur between patients and providers—in other words, what is done to the patient—are considered process measures. Preventive care activities such as immunizations and prenatal care are examples of process measures. As discussed in Chapter 8, CMS initiated its quality reporting initiative using condition-specific inpatient process measures. Changes in clinical status—in other words, what happens to the patient—are considered outcome measures. Healthcare-associated infections are examples of outcome measures.

Managers may also classify measures into the following categories set forth by the Institute of Medicine (2001b, 7) in *Envisioning the National Health Care Quality Report*:

- Safety refers to avoiding injuries to patients from care that is intended to help them.
- Effectiveness refers to providing services based on scientific knowledge to all who could benefit and refraining from providing services to those not likely to benefit (avoiding overuse and misuse).
- Patient centeredness refers to healthcare that establishes a partnership among practitioners, patients, and their families (when appropriate) to ensure that decisions respect patients' wants, needs, and preferences and that patients have the education and support they require to make decisions and participate in their own care.
- Timeliness refers to obtaining needed care and minimizing delays in getting that care.

A varied set of measures that are vertically and horizontally aligned, combined with a systematic way of analyzing and communicating information gleaned from the measures, aid managers in identifying patterns across parts of the system, provide clues about system structures, and help ensure that one area of performance is not unintentionally excelling at the expense of another. Performance indicators throughout the organization should reflect the common direction and priorities defined by the organization's mission, vision, and business strategy. A comprehensive performance management measurement system should also ensure coordination of activities to minimize the duplication of collecting, reporting, and analyzing efforts.

Analyze Process and System Performance

Process performance is based on several concepts and principles. Process requirements, also referred to as the "voice of the customer," define what is needed from the process; process capability, also referred to as the "voice of the process," is what the process can deliver; process measurement quantifies the voice of the process; process behavior charts illustrate the difference between the voice of the customer and the voice of the process; and process improvement helps align process capability with process requirements.

Process Requirements

Process requirements are the outputs the manager expects the process to deliver. In health services organizations, process requirements may be considered from the perspectives of patients, internal customers, other stakeholders, and the market in general. Chapter 7 describes the various sources of process requirements. Clinical studies, guidelines, and practice standards are also sources of process requirements in health services. Organizations operating from the mature end of the quality continuum understand that customer, stakeholder, and market requirements are the foundation for and drive all work performed by the organization.

Process Capability and Process Measurement

Process capability is what the process is able to deliver (Wheeler 2000). The run chart in Exhibit 9.9 shows a change in process capability when the hand hygiene rates gradually yet steadily increased after the intervention. Every process has a built-in capacity to deliver outputs within a defined range. Process requirements guide the selection of metrics to quantify the process capability. Consider the example of a hospitalized patient experiencing pain. The voice of the customer (process requirement) in this case is a consistent, timely response when requesting assistance. The voice of the process (process capability) is how long it takes for the patient to receive assistance when requested. The voice of the process may be measured in minutes from the time the patient asks for help to the time someone responds to the request. Collecting the response times for a defined period of time—say for a day—provides insight about the process capability. Exhibit 10.12 displays sample response-time data for two different hospitals with the minutes on the x-axis and number of requests on the y-axis.

Patients in Hospital 1 will receive help within 4 to 16 minutes and those in Hospital 2 within 2 to 6 minutes. The range of response times reflects the process capability at each hospital: the larger the range in minutes, the less dependable the process; the lower the range in minutes, the more dependable and predictable the process. In this example, Hospital 2 responds more quickly and more consistently than Hospital 1 to a patient's request for

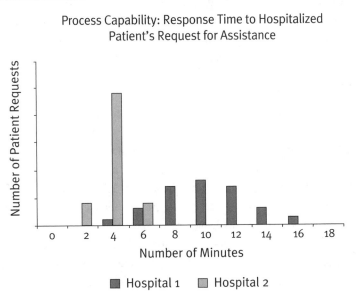

Process Capability: Response Time to Hospitalized Patient's Request for Assistance

Number of Patient Requests

Number of Minutes

■ Hospital 1   ■ Hospital 2

EXHIBIT 10.12
Response Times Frequency Distribution Bar Graph

EXHIBIT 10.13

Response
Times
Frequency
Distribution
Line Graph

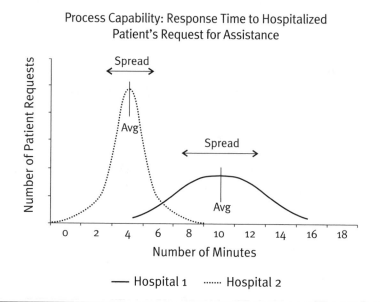

Process Capability: Response Time to Hospitalized
Patient's Request for Assistance

assistance. The voice of the Hospital 1 process shows a process designed in a manner that delivers inconsistent rather than dependable results. Adding training, working harder, or setting new goals will be ineffective strategies to improve the output of this process. The process delivers outputs within the range of its capability and will change only if the process itself is changed.

The frequency distribution may also be plotted as a line graph like the one shown in Exhibit 10.13. Displayed this way, the response times resemble normal distribution curves. Several calculations may be derived from the distribution, including a measure of central tendency such as a mean or an average and a measure of spread or distance from the average such as a standard deviation. When the process is carried out, performance is expected to fall within the area under the curve.

Process Behavior Charts

While a frequency distribution shows process performance for a defined time period, process performance may be plotted and tracked over time. Turning the frequency distribution on its side forms the basic process behavior chart, with the increments of time on the x-axis and the units of performance on the y-axis. This simple rotation to the frequency distributions in Exhibit 10.13 is shown in Exhibit 10.14. Three horizontal lines are added, representing the average and the upper and lower range of values.

Plotting the average response times (e.g., daily averages for a week, weekly averages for a month) provides additional insight about the process capability, its average level of performance, and the amount of variation in the process over time (Exhibit 10.15).

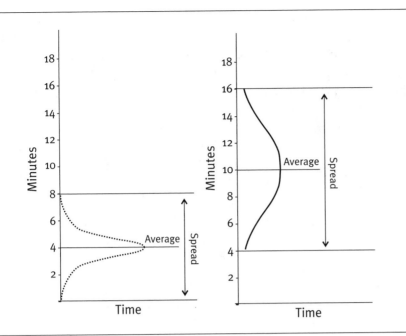

EXHIBIT 10.14
Converting the Frequency Distribution to a Process Behavior Chart

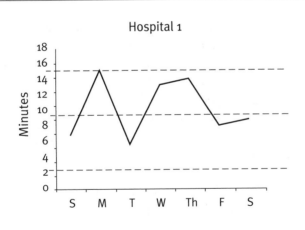

EXHIBIT 10.15
Simple Process Behavior Charts of Average Daily Response Times for Hospitalized Patients' Requests for Assistance

A manager must be able to recognize the two types of variation illus-trated by process behavior charts. **Random variation**, also referred to as noise or common cause variation, is the natural variation present in the process (Carey and Lloyd 2001). For example, in the Hospital 1 chart in Exhibit 10.15, the process did not suddenly deteriorate from Monday to Tuesday. The daily change simply represents the amount of random variation inherent in this process.

Assignable variation, also referred to as a signal or special cause variation, indicates that something irregular (i.e., not inherent to the process) has occurred (Carey and Lloyd 2001). The manager can distinguish random variation as those points that lie within the boundaries of the upper and lower control limits. Assignable or special cause variation is present when the manager sees any of the following situations (Wheeler 2000):

- A value that is above the upper control limit or below the lower control limit
- Three to four successive values that lie closer to the control limits than to the mean
- Eight or more consecutive points that lie on the same side of the mean

For example, in the Hospital 2 chart in Exhibit 10.15, the average response time on Friday is well above the upper limit. This is an example of a one-time irregularity, such as unexpected last-minute staff sick calls leaving the department short-handed for part of the day.

The reason a manager must be able to distinguish between random and assignable variation is that she will need to respond differently depending on the type of variation present. A manager cannot do anything to change the amount of random variation exhibited by the process except to change, redesign, or improve the underlying process itself. On the other hand, assignable variation results from a distinct cause that warrants investigation by the manager. A one-time, assignable variation may be traced to its cause and explained. Assignable variation, represented by a series of points, is a clue that an intentional or unintentional change in the process has occurred. One expects to see a change in process capability after an improvement intervention. The desired impact is more consistent and predictable processes, which result in a narrowing range of random variation and a shift in the average level of performance in a favorable direction.

When reading a process behavior chart, remember the underlying curve and its measures of central tendency and spread. Process behavior charts may be designed by establishing boundaries at plus or minus three standard deviations from the mean (capturing how the process performs about 99 percent of the time) or they may be designed by establishing boundaries at plus or minus two standard deviations from the mean (capturing how the process performs about 95 percent of the time). A detailed explanation of the statistical calculations of process behavior charts is beyond the scope of this text. Readers are encouraged to consult a statistician or management engineer and refer to the references for more technical guidance on constructing process behavior charts.

Process Improvement

Tools for analyzing and improving processes are discussed in Chapter 9. Managers must also consider that, because of the interrelationships among the parts of the system, improvement in complex systems will not likely result in straightforward cause-and-effect relationships as seen in a controlled research study. Process behavior charts provide important clues to system, as well as process, behavior. As Wheeler states (2000, 79);

- The voice of the customer defines what you want from a system.
- The voice of the process defines what you will get from the system.
- Management's job is to work to bring the voice of the process into alignment with the voice of the customer.

Consider the example introduced in Chapter 9 about improving hand hygiene. On first glance, hand washing might appear to be straightforward; however, numerous factors contribute to consistent and successful practice, as illustrated in the simple cause-and-effect diagram (see Exhibit 9.7). Improving one of these causes can increase compliance a little; however, a problem with multiple causes requires a multifaceted improvement plan. For example, the World Health Organization (WHO) endorses a combination of interventions (Exhibit 10.16) to improve the hand-hygiene compliance of health services workers.

System Change: ensuring that the necessary infrastructure is in place to allow healthcare workers to practice hand hygiene.

Training/Education: providing regular training on the importance of hand hygiene, based on the "My 5 Moments for Hand Hygiene" approach, and the correct procedures for hand rubbing and hand washing, to all healthcare workers.

Evaluation and Feedback: monitoring hand-hygiene practices and infrastructure, along with related perceptions and knowledge among healthcare workers, while providing performance and results feedback to staff.

Reminders in the Workplace: prompting and reminding healthcare workers about the importance of hand hygiene and about the appropriate indications and procedures for performing it.

Institutional Safety Climate: creating an environment and the perceptions that facilitate awareness-raising about patient safety issues while guaranteeing consideration of hand hygiene improvement as a high priority at all levels.

EXHIBIT 10.16
WHO Hand-Hygiene Recommendations

Source: World Health Organization. 2009. *A Guide to the Implementation of the WHO Multimodal Hand Hygiene Improvement Strategy.* Retrieved 10/31/10 from: www.who.int/gpsc/5may/tools/en/. © World Health Orgabnization 2009. All rights reserved.

EXHIBIT 10.17

Three-Year
Hand-Hygiene
Compliance
Rates

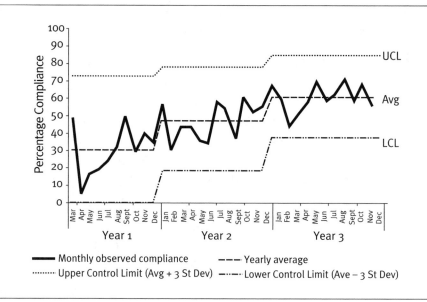

Implementing the WHO guidelines involves improving multiple processes and engaging multiple stakeholders and departments throughout an organization on a continual basis. The guidelines also reflect the systems lessons on goals discussed in Chapter 6: "In complex situations, we must almost always avoid focusing on just one element and pursuing only one goal; instead, we must pursue several goals at once" (Dorner 1996, 64). While individual interventions should be monitored for successful implementation, the resulting change in system behavior depends not only on the individual interventions but also on the interdependencies among the interventions. Exhibit 10.17 illustrates one organization's experience with continuous attention to and improvement of its multifaceted hand-hygiene initiative. The process behavior chart tracks system behavior over three years measured by hand-hygiene compliance rates. One sees an improvement of the average compliance rate per year and the narrowing of the range, indicating more predictable and dependable behavior in the direction of 100 percent compliance.

Performance Management Measures and the Quality Continuum

Managers must recognize the difference between managing the indicators and managing performance. Although a manager may successfully report the performance indicators required by internal and external stakeholders, he may still not be successfully managing his organization. For example, a hospital may demonstrate above the national average on the CMS Surgical Care Improvement Project Process of Care Measures, such as administering timely prophylactic antibiotics (HHS 2010), yet still be plagued with surgeries not starting on time. The same hospital may consistently document the pre-procedure time-out required by the National Patient Safety Goals (The Joint Commission 2010e), yet still experience excessive overtime pay and delays in transferring patients to an inpatient bed.

Managers must see performance—not simply performance indicators—as the end result of their efforts. According to the Baldrige Performance Excellence Program Health Care Criteria (NIST 2011, 1), "measurement, analysis and knowledge-management are critical to the effective management of your organization and to a fact-based, knowledge-driven system for improving healthcare and operational performance" and "serve as a foundation for the performance management system." In other words, measurement is essential to managing and improving organizational performance and results.

An organization's use of performance management measures provides clues about their progress along the quality continuum. As illustrated in Exhibit 10.18, those embarking on new or early efforts are on the far left of the continuum and are lacking data important to the mission. Those who are experienced in their efforts, shown on the far right, collect data that reflect key business requirements, demonstrate performance from key business processes, and monitor progress on strategic action plans (NIST 2011).

The performance measurement continuum in Exhibit 10.18 references comparative data. The purpose of using comparative data is to better understand one's own organizations' performance within the context of how other similar organizations and the industry in general are performing. Comparing data can lead to identifying best practices and aid in revealing systemic structures. In recent years, availability of and access to comparative data in healthcare have greatly improved. Exhibit 10.19 provides data sources that managers may use in comparing performance data.

Summary

Traditional linear approaches to measuring and analyzing performance have limitations when applied to complex systems. This chapter offers lessons for managers to assist them in better understanding and improving system behavior, including preserving the data's context, bundling and unbundling data, understanding the user's purpose of the data, differentiating types of measures, selecting a balanced set of measures, and analyzing process and system behavior with process behavior charts. This chapter also illustrates the role of performance measurement along the quality continuum and provides resources for managers to find comparative data.

EXHIBIT 10.18

The Quality
Continuum in
Performance
Measurement

Results are not reported for any areas of importance to the accomplishment of your organization's mission.	Results are reported for a few areas of importance to the accomplishment of your organization's mission.	Results are reported for many areas of importance to the accomplishment of your organization's mission.	Organizational performance results are reported for most key patient and stakeholder, market, and process requirements.	Organizational performance results are reported for most key patient and stakeholder, market, process, and action plan requirements.	Organizational performance results fully address key patient and stakeholder, market, process, and action plan requirements.
Comparative information is not reported.	Little or no comparative information is reported.	Early stages of obtaining comparative information are evident.	Some current performance levels have been evaluated against relevant comparisons and/or benchmarks and show areas of good relative performance.	Many to most trends and current performance levels have been evaluated against relevant comparisons and/or benchmarks and show areas of leadership and very good relative performance.	Evidence of industry and benchmark leadership is demonstrated in many areas.
Trend data either are not reported or show mainly adverse trends.	Some trend data are reported, with some adverse trends evident.	Some trend data are reported, and a majority of the trends presented are beneficial.	Beneficial trends are evident in areas of importance to the accomplishment of your organization's mission.	Beneficial trends have been sustained over time in most areas of importance to the accomplishment of your organization's mission.	Beneficial trends have been sustained over time in all areas of importance to the accomplishment of your organization's mission.
There are no organizational performance results and/or poor results in areas reported.	A few organizational performance results are reported, and early good performance levels are evident.	Good organizational performance levels are reported for some areas of importance.	Good organizational performance levels are reported for most areas of importance.	Good to excellent organizational performance levels are reported for most areas of importance.	Excellent organizational performance levels are reported.

Early efforts ——————————————————————————▶ Mature efforts

Source: Adapted from National Institute of Standards and Technology (2011).

EXHIBIT 10.19
Sources of
Comparative
Data

Patient Satisfaction

Consumer Assessment of Healthcare Providers and Systems	www.cahps.ahrq.gov
Hospital Compare	www.hospitalcompare.hhs.gov

Health Plans

National Committee for Quality Assurance (NCQA)	www.ncqa.org

Population Data

Centers for Disease Control and Prevention: Data and Statistics site	www.cdc.gov/DataStatistics/
State health departments	
AHRQ (National Healthcare Quality Report and National Healthcare Disparities Report)	www.ahrq.gov/qual/
KFF Statehealthfacts.org	www.statehealthfacts.org/
KFF Globalhealthfacts.org	www.globalhealthfacts.org/

Clinical Data

Disease-specific registries	
The Joint Commission Quality Check	www.qualitycheck.org
Hospital Compare (disease-specific clinical indicators)	www.hospitalcompare.hhs.gov
Nursing Home Quality Initiative with link to Nursing Home Compare (long-term and short-stay indicators)	www.medicare.gov/NHCompare
Home Health Quality Initiative with link to Home Health Compare (Home Health Outcome and Assessment Information Set or OASIS indicators)	www.medicare.gov/HHCompare

Comparative Practices

Baldrige Performance Excellence Program Awardees	www.nist.gov/baldrige/ award_recipients/index.cfm

Exercise

Background: This exercise further explores the principle about data and complex systems discussed in this chapter: "Graphs reveal interesting structures present in the data" (Wheeler 2000, 14, 79).

Objective: Evaluate graphic presentations of data and select the one that provides the most valuable feedback about the system's behavior.

Instructions:

As the manager of an emergency department (ED), you are faced with the challenge of improving flow and better matching your staffing plan to patient demand. Like the mammography center manager in this chapter, your monthly reports from the finance department present the ED's volume statistics in a spreadsheet according to this month, last month, year to date, and the same month, previous year. You decide to graph the data. You experiment with the data and come up with the following three graphs using the exact same data. Select the graph that provides you with the most insight and explain why you chose that graph.

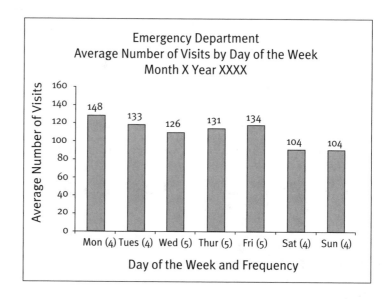

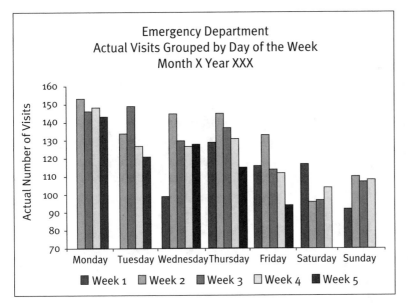

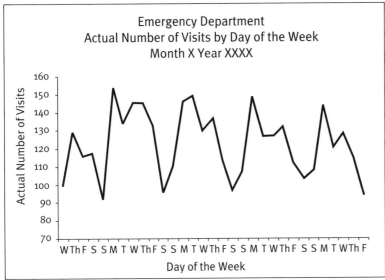

Companion Readings

Neely, A., and M. A. Najjar. 2006. "Management Learning: Not Management Control: The True Role of Performance Measurement?" *California Management Review* 48 (3): 101–14.

Wheeler, D. J. 2000. *Understanding Variation: The Key to Managing Chaos,* 2nd ed. Knoxville, TN: SPC Press.

Web Resources

AHRQ Quality Indicators website: www.qualityindicators.ahrq.gov/
National Quality Measures Clearing House: www.qualitymeasures.ahrq.gov/

FOSTERING TEAMWORK: BELOW-THE-WATERLINE CONSIDERATIONS

Learning Objectives

After completing this chapter you should be able to:

- compare mental models about teams and their role in team effectiveness and
- describe the importance of purposeful team design on organizational results.

As the department managers at Hospital A sit around the conference table, their minds are elsewhere. One is reviewing financial reports, one is in and out of the room answering phone calls, and they all are intermittently reading and answering messages on their smart phones. The administrator keeps talking, oblivious to the indifference and apathy of the people in the room. Because attendance weighs heavily in the manager's performance appraisal, all managers attend the monthly management team meetings. According to anyone who is asked, the meetings are "a waste of time, but you have to go."

The administrator at Hospital B starts by reviewing the purpose of the monthly management team meeting: to provide a forum for information sharing, learning, and collaborative problem solving and improvement. The team consists of the managers within the administrator's scope of responsibility, and the human resources, quality, and financial consultants dedicated to her service line. Each participant is leafing through the agenda packet as the administrator reviews the items that will be discussed during the next two hours: "First, each manager will summarize his or her performance indicators for the month. The summary graphs for each department are in your packet, and so is the entire service line report. Please be sure to point out the positive trends and alert us to potential problems. Second on the agenda is a brief presentation from Manager A about the results of a recent improvement effort and what his team learned from the process. Finally, Manager B will summarize the important points from the conference she attended last week. Does anyone need to add anything to the agenda?" At the conclusion of the meeting, the managers are still milling around the room, asking each other questions, laughing together, and competitively joking about whose performance statistics have shown the most improvement this year.

In both of these examples, highly paid managerial employees are brought together regularly for a meeting. However, the yield from each meeting differs. Predictably, the overall yield from each manager and from the service line as a whole also differs. The collective intelligence of the organization is often an underrecognized variable in the productivity equation, especially when applied to knowledge work like healthcare.

The ability to effectively design and manage teams is an essential management skill. The published literature already offers managers a wealth of information about teams, so this chapter does not review or summarize that information. This chapter does, however, explore some practical team strategies related to the specific concepts described in this book.

Team Design

Team
a number of persons associated together in work or activity (Merriam-Webster Dictionary Online 2010c)

The dictionary defines a **team** as a number of persons associated together in work or activity (Merriam-Webster Dictionary Online 2010c). Many types of teams are seen in health services organizations. Teams may be based on a function, such as research teams or management teams; teams may be based on a professional specialty, such as physician teams or informatics teams; and teams may be based in a department or division, such as oncology teams or chronic care teams. Teams may comprise specialties within a single discipline, across disciplines, across departments, or across organizations. Clinical teams may work in an environment focused on interventions that are accomplished within hours, such as an operating room team, or they may work in an environment focused on interventions that are accomplished in weeks or months, such as a rehabilitation team. Team membership may be fluid and change on a daily basis; team membership may be stable for the duration of a project.

The term "team" carries with it many meanings, perceptions, and approaches, depending on one's frame of reference. Just as Chapter 1 discusses the value of a shared definition of quality, managers must ensure a shared definition of team, team roles, expectations, and communication if teams are to execute their responsibilities in a safe, effective, and quality manner. Consider the "simple" analogy of a sports team. A brief comparison of four different types of college sports teams is illustrated in Exhibit 11.1.

One can quickly see the numerous opportunities for misunderstandings and misinterpretations unless the simple sports analogy is further defined by the type of game being played. Team members may have the same title (i.e., center) but different roles depending on which game they are playing (football or basketball). Some teams are totally dependent on each other minute by minute to win a game (football, basketball, volleyball); some teams win by accumulating wins by individuals (golf, tennis). The term "point" has a range of values; some teams win games, some win matches; some teams

Type of Team	How Many Team Members Play Together at Once?	What Are the Team Member Roles?	How Does One Measure Success?	How Does the Team Win?	EXHIBIT 11.1
Football	11 players on the field at one time	Backs, safety, center, tackle, end, receiver	Touchdown: 7 points Field goal: 3 points	Most points	Comparison of College Sports Teams
Basketball	5 people on the court at one time	Guard, forward, center	Field goal: 2 points or 3 points Free throw: 1 point at time	Most points	
Golf	Team competes on an individual level	Golfer	Strokes	Fewest strokes	
Volleyball	Depending on the type of volleyball: 1, 2, 5, 6, or 8	Setter, hitter, blocker	Points	Game: first team to reach 15 or 25; must win by 2 points Match: team that wins best of 5 games	
Tennis	Singles: 1 player Doubles: 2 players	Player	Love = 0 points Point = 15 points Advantage	Game: 45 points; must win by 2 points Set: best of 3 or best of 5 games	

win with the most points, some with the fewest; some teams must reach a defined score, with some teams the winning score can vary. Imagine players from each of the sports placed together on a unique five-person team and asked to play a new game for which there are no rules. A comparable scenario often plays out in health services organizations. The diversity of the health services workforce and the dynamic complexity inherent in the industry beg for a common, shared understanding of the concept of "team" and how it is operationalized in one's specific organization.

Effective teams do not just happen; they are thoughtfully and purposefully designed. The following sequence of questions should be asked any time a manager is considering a team approach on any level, whether for a management team, a project team, a care delivery team, or an improvement team.

1. What is the purpose of the team (e.g., activity, process, function)?
2. What is the ideal, step-by-step process or approach to achieve that purpose?
3. What is the most appropriate structure to support and carry out that process? (Structure includes how people are organized to carry out the process, how roles are defined, and how the roles interact with each other.)
4. How does the team define and measure success?

When the two meeting examples at the beginning of the chapter are critiqued according to these questions, one discovers that the management team meetings in Hospital A do not have a purpose or a defined process. Although the structure is defined, without addressing the first two questions, this structure has little impact on manager effectiveness and, in turn, on departmental and organizational performance. In Hospital B, the purpose is clearly defined as providing a forum for information sharing, learning, collaborative problem solving, and improvement. The step-by-step process to achieve this purpose is a defined agenda at each meeting that includes discussing performance indicators, sharing successes and individuals' learning, and communicating organizational information from administrators to managers, managers to administrators, and managers to managers. The team members include not only the managers but also a financial officer, a human resources consultant, and a quality department staff member, and the entire team is assigned to the service line. These additional team members assist with compiling the performance data, generating management reports, and answering data-related questions at the meetings. Guest speakers are invited to address special topics. Department and service line performance indicators are clearly defined, measured, reported, and analyzed. Not only do the managers in this service line demonstrate a high level of individual performance and satisfaction, but overall the service line also consistently demonstrates the highest level of relative improvement year after year compared to other service lines in the organization.

Mental Models Affecting Team Design

The manager's mental models and the organization's context (see chapters 3 and 5) influence how teams are defined, designed, and employed in an organization. Historically, when a physician entered the hospital unit, nurses offered their chairs to the physician because the nurses held lower positions in the organizational and professional hierarchies governing power, status, and authority. Remnants of this tradition (e.g., deferring to someone higher in the hierarchy, ordering about someone lower in the hierarchy) may still be seen in how health services organizations approach teams, teamwork, or lack thereof. Helmreich writes of an instance when "a distinguished neuro-surgeon persists in operating on the wrong side of a woman's brain, in spite of vague protests by a resident who is aware of the error" (Helmreich 1997, 67). Mental models about authority can influence communication within team settings and, in turn, the quality of clinical outcomes. If the mental model guiding this operating team is that the surgeon knows best and no one challenges the surgeon, the resulting wrong-site surgery is not surprising.

Academic centers are steeped in traditions based on multiple and parallel hierarchies. For example, novel ideas from junior and/or non-tenured faculty may be dismissed simply because of their position in the hierarchy rather than the merit of the idea. In the academic medical center, the CEO and the administrative team occupy the top positions in the management hierarchy, and frontline supervisors occupy the bottom. The department chairs are at the top of the medical staff hierarchy, and the interns or medical students are at the bottom. Physicians, followed by nurses, are at the top of the professional hierarchy, whereas other professionals (e.g., social workers, occupational therapists) all hold nondescript places lower in the hierarchy. Physicians and nurses hold the top spots in the jobs hierarchy, and the hourly manual laborers (e.g., environmental services and food service workers) are designated to the lower spots. Although each group performs its respective duties in a competent manner, the hierarchies foster a fragmented approach to patient care. For example, physician teams typically make their morning patient rounds while nurses are occupied with the change-of-shift report. As a result, the nurses and physicians caring for the same patients rarely talk to each other during the course of day-to-day patient care.

From this traditional mental model, the hospital can demonstrate many examples of quality improvement team projects; however, its teams tend to have an exclusive makeup (e.g., physician teams or nurse teams). Although departments such as the laboratory attempt on numerous occasions to create improvement teams with a mix of different providers, they have little success in crossing the rigid boundaries of the professional and job hierarchies in the organization. Although the hospital is able to identify many improvement teams, only a few examples of teamwork across and within these hierarchies can be seen.

Another way to view teams in health services organizations is from a clinical microsystem mental model. Although the concept of high-performance work teams is not new in other industries (Hanlan 2004), the application of these lessons to the health services delivery setting is relatively recent. Nelson and colleagues (2007) have studied high-performing, frontline clinical teams in various healthcare settings and offer insights into success factors for designing a clinical microsystem to enhance quality outcomes and patient safety. A clinical **microsystem** is defined as a "a small group of people who work together on a regular basis to provide care to discrete

Microsystem (clinical)
"[a] small group of people who work together on a regular basis to provide care to discrete subpopulations of patients . . . a microsystem is the local milieu in which patients, providers, support staff, information, and processes converge for the purpose of providing care to individual people to meet their health needs" (Nelson et al. 2007)

subpopulations of patients . . . a microsystem is the local milieu in which patients, providers, support staff, information, and processes converge for the purpose of providing care to individual people to meet their health needs" (Nelson et al. 2007, 7). High-performing microsystems are characterized by

> constancy of purpose, investment in improvement, alignment of role and training for efficiency and staff satisfaction, interdependence of care team to meet patient needs, integration of information and technology into work flows, ongoing measurement of outcomes, supportiveness of the larger organization, and connection to the community to enhance care delivery and extend influence. (Nelson et al. 2007, 14)

Upon closer examination, one sees that these characteristics result from intentional role and team design.

Because leadership sets direction for the organization (see chapters 5 and 6), leaders' mental models can shape the organization's direction, context, and operating values. Mental models about medical errors can shape operating values related to teams and teamwork. A mental model of "individual vigilance is the best protection against medical errors" would likely lead to teamwork that resembles a tennis team or a golf team; however, a mental model that accepts errors as "inevitable" (Helmreich, Merritt, and Wilhelm 1999) would lead to team design that resembles football, basketball, or volleyball, where team members have defined roles, plays are planned and coordinated in advance, team members guard and protect each other, and members step up to save a play if something goes wrong.

The mental model of accepting errors as inevitable provides the foundation for the team approach referred to as **crew resource management** or CRM. CRM started in aviation and recently has been making its way to health services; "CRM can be seen as a set of error countermeasures with three lines of defense. The first, naturally, is the avoidance of error. The second is trapping incipient errors before they are committed. The third and last is mitigating the consequences of those errors which occur and are not trapped" (Helmreich, Merritt, and Wilhelm 1999, 27). In the absence of the belief that errors are inevitable, team design may lack the built-in lines of defense integral to safe operation and execution (see Exhibit 4.5).

Mental Models About Talents and Differences

Many managers and employees may prefer agreement and harmony; however, diverse perspectives supply the essential elements of creative tension and have been credited with innovation and improvement. "Innovate or fall behind: the competitive imperative for virtually all businesses today is that simple. Achieving it is hard, however, because innovation takes place when different

---

Crew resource management (CRM)

team approach that accepts errors as inevitable and includes "a set of error countermeasures with three lines of defense. The first, naturally, is the avoidance of error. The second is trapping incipient errors before they are committed. The third and last is mitigating the consequences of those errors which occur and are not trapped" (Helmreich, Merritt, and Wilhelm 1999, 27) ideas, perceptions, and ways of processing and judging information collide. That, in turn, often requires collaboration among various players who see the world in inherently different ways" (Leonard and Straus 1997, 111).

Although diverse perspectives serve a role in creative tension and foster innovation, they also create fertile ground for accidental adversaries (Chapter 3), conflict, and team breakdowns. Managers are challenged to find tools and approaches that enable them to take advantage of differing perspectives while maintaining effective interpersonal relationships within teams and employee groups. How can managers promote friction among ideas while minimizing friction among people?

Numerous frameworks are available to help managers understand and appreciate individuals and their differences. Although the taxonomy may vary, each framework defines groups on the basis of common patterns. Studies of large numbers of individuals have resulted in the identification of patterns in their preferences, predispositions, temperaments, learning styles, and strengths. These patterns have been organized and labeled according to various frameworks, including the Myers-Briggs Type Indicator, the Keirsey Temperament Sorter, Human Dynamics, and the StrengthsFinder. Specific descriptions of these frameworks are not provided in this book, but readers are encouraged to further explore them; see the Web Resources for this chapter.

When these different frameworks are studied as a group, patterns begin to emerge. First, the frameworks recognize that individuals bring differences with them to the workplace. The frameworks identify, categorize, and explain those differences and provide a concrete and systematic means of recognizing, describing, and understanding the differences. The frameworks also provide a common language and approach for managers and teams within the organization to understand, appreciate, and address differences in the workplace in a positive way. When two of these frameworks—the Myers-Briggs Type Indicator and Human Dynamics—are studied together, some global, cross-cutting dichotomies may be seen. These include the following dualities: internal and external, practical and creative, data oriented and relationship oriented, concrete and conceptual, linear and lateral, and spontaneous and structured. Managers should begin to look for how they express these global dichotomies and how their employees and teams express these dichotomies, as the dualities influence preferences regarding leadership, communication, learning, and client interactions. Managing the interface of these dichotomies, rather than avoiding or falling victim to them, will enable managers to enhance the effectiveness of operational working teams and improvement project teams.

The manager's responsibility is to select the desired lens (i.e., manage the context; see Chapter 5) through which individuals within the organization and the organization as a whole will view their work and workplace. A lens that views differences as complementary talents may result in synergy and success, while a lens that views differences as opposing perspectives may result in conflict, breakdowns, and mediocrity.

For example, as client volumes increased, a department grew from 5 employees to 20 almost overnight. When there were only five employees, the department functioned like a close-knit family. Yet when new employees came on board, they found themselves thrown into the work with little time to assimilate into the culture and style of the team. For the first time, the department appointed a supervisor to oversee the team, and not long after that the complaints started: "The supervisor never follows through on anything"; "A certain employee is not carrying her load"; or "The supervisor is all talk and no action."

This department inadvertently set up an accidental adversaries situation between the supervisor and the staff. In Chapter 3, the term "accidental adversaries" is used in relation to double-loop learning. Accidental adversaries, which result from differences in styles, learning preferences, and personality types, can be a common and unrecognized source of conflict in all kinds of teams.

When the employees in this department took the Myers-Briggs Type Indicator test, the results were illuminating. Of the 20 department employees, 18 were *sensing* types. They prefer the concrete, real, factual, structured, and tangible here and now; they become impatient with the abstract and mistrust intuition. Two of the employees, including the supervisor, were *intuitive* types. They preferred possibilities, theories, invention, and the new; they enjoyed discussions characterized by spontaneous leaps of intuition, and they tended to leave out or neglect details (Myers, Kirby, and Myers 1998). In this department, the supervisor inherently functioned in a manner that was opposite to the rest of the department's way of functioning. As a result, misunderstandings, misperceptions, and communication breakdowns became common.

When these differences were understood, the department could put into place specific processes and systems (which were not necessary when there were only a few employees) to minimize the potential breakdowns. For example, a standing agenda at staff meetings helped the supervisor stay on task and avoid getting sidetracked. A bulletin board, e-mail messages, and a shared network drive were used to ensure that current and complete information about departmental issues was available to everyone. A human resources performance measurement system was put into place to provide a factual base for evaluating individual productivity and workload.

By understanding and implementing processes designed to meet the differing information and communication needs of the sensing and intuitive types, the department was able to avert further conflict and misunderstanding and focus employees' energy on productive work rather than on perceived supervisory deficiencies.

Mental Models About Improvement or Project Teams

Assembling the Team

For an improvement project team, team composition (the number and identity of the members) and meeting frequency and duration should be guided by the purpose and team processes for the improvement effort. The questions that should be asked include:

- What knowledge is required to understand the process and design the actual improvement intervention(s)?
- How should the team be designed to support the processes needed to accomplish implementation within the project constraints?

Focusing on early adopters has been shown to be an effective strategy to get individuals to adopt an innovation. Once approximately 5 to 20 percent of a group has successfully adopted a new process, adoption by the rest of the required group progresses rapidly (Rogers 1995). According to the Myers-Briggs Type Indicator, approximately 68 percent of the population expresses a personality type that is resistant to change, and 32 percent express a type that is accepting of change (Myers, Kirby, and Myers 1998; Smith 2000). Within the two groups exists an entire continuum of resistance and acceptance. Typically, early adopters of innovations fall into specific Myers-Briggs types.

What does a manager do when faced with implementing improvements when few early adopters are in the employee pool? This was the case for a manager who needed to obtain rapid buy-in for a large change effort in a department composed mostly of people with resistant personality types. The manager chose a strategy involving a 40-member improvement team, which represented about 25 percent of the total department staff and included formal and informal leaders in the department. Although most of these 40 people fell into the "resistant" group, by involving them earlier rather than later in the process, the manager not only engaged those who readily accepted change but also simultaneously cultivated the critical mass of the resistant types needed to support implementation of the improvements. In this way, the speed with which the improvements were adopted and implemented throughout the entire department was greatly enhanced (Kelly 1998).

Just as managers use human resources practices that promote matching an employee's traits with the requirements of the job, managers may also match employees with the various roles and stages required in a change or improvement process. Problems in group processes tend to arise from a mismatch between a process stage and an individual rather than from problems inherent in the individuals themselves. Purposefully engaging individuals at the appropriate time in the process and offering support and requesting patience during other times can enhance the team's and the manager's effectiveness.

A team member favoring a concrete pattern may get frustrated with creating a vision, although he will be essential in determining the logistics of the implementation. Someone with an interpersonal or relational pattern can be on the alert for any employee issues related to the changes. An employee with a pattern of seeing the big picture will be invaluable in identifying unintended consequences. A team member who is detail oriented can be an ideal choice for monitoring progress and ensuring follow-through; another member who is action oriented can make sure the team gets moving.

Meeting Schedules and Frequency

Typical meetings are held weekly, biweekly, or monthly, and they generally last one to two hours. Some of the challenges associated with this approach in health services organizations include clinical providers not being able to get away from daily patient care duties, team members arriving late because of other competing responsibilities, the need to devote portions of the meeting to updating team members, and dwindling interest as the process drags on.

Consider an alternative approach. If managers use a systematic method for approaching improvements, they will begin to get a sense for the total team time required for an improvement effort. For example, a team may take about 40 hours to complete the various phases of an improvement project. If the improvement effort is constrained by time or dollars, the team is faced with increasing its own productivity or reducing its own cycle time. With this in mind, the 40 hours of time may be distributed in a variety of ways other than in one-to-two-hour segments. For example, ten four-hour meetings or five eight-hour meetings may better meet the needs of a particular project. The meetings may occur once a week for ten weeks, twice a week for five weeks, or every day for one week. Based on the particular work environment, a strategy may be selected that balances project-team productivity, daily operational capacity and requirements, the scope of the desired improvement, and project deadlines.

A concentrated team meeting schedule has several advantages:

- It demonstrates the organization's or management's commitment to change.
- It saves duplication and rework associated with bringing everyone up to speed at each meeting.
- It establishes traction by contributing to the elements of creative tension.
- It reduces the cycle time from concept to implementation.
- It forces managers and teams out of the "firefighting" mentality into one of purposely fixing not just the symptoms of problems but also the underlying problems themselves.

Decision Making

Consensus is a widespread approach to decision making in which the team seeks to find a proposal acceptable enough that all members can support it (Scholtes, Joiner, and Streibel 2003). Seeking consensus may, however, reduce decisions to the lowest common denominator (Wheatley 1994). In a team comprising primarily concrete, practical, linear-thinking members, how likely is it that an idea posed by the one creative, conceptual team member will gain enough acceptance to be considered a possible solution to a problem? Or conversely, on a team of creative, conceptual innovators who are quickly moving forward on an idea without regard for the practical considerations of implementation, how likely will it be that they embrace the input from the one concrete, practical, linear-thinking team member? In either case, the result will be less than optimal. The best result (i.e., improvement intervention) in these two circumstances may come from listening to the "outlier"; perhaps that team member's perspective best matches the requirements of the decision at hand. Using decision criteria is an alternative to consensus. Using criteria does not imply that a team is not accountable for supporting a decision once it is made; it suggests that decisions will more likely take a diverse perspective into consideration. For example, in one improvement effort, the criteria for pursuing an improvement idea include the following (Kelly 1998):

- Does it fit within the goal of the effort?
- Does it meet customer requirements?
- Does it meet regulatory/accreditation requirements?
- Does it remain consistent with the department's/organization's purpose?
- Does it support the vision?
- Does it demonstrate consistency with quality principles?

In this case, team members are expected to question and challenge an idea, and if an idea meets the criteria the team can pursue it further, confident that the idea is sound. Although all team members may not completely understand the idea at the time, much time is saved from trying to explain something that is not readily understandable given the individual natures of the team members.

Tools for Effective Teams

The manager's responsibility is to ensure the team has the resources, tools, and leadership support to be successful (see Chapter 1; Kelly and Short 2006).

Human Resource Tools

Chapter 1 discusses how managers today must be keenly aware of the way human resources issues affect their ability not only to support teamwork but also to promote quality patient outcomes and cost effectiveness. An effective team design requires appropriate human resources to be executed effectively. Consider the impact of nurse staffing on inpatient outcomes. A growing body of evidence links physician, nurse, and pharmacist staffing with patient outcomes in the hospital setting (Pronovost et al. 2002; Horn and Jacobi 2006; Clarke 2007; Clarke and Donaldson 2008; Lopez et al. 2009; Harrison and Curran 2009). For example, levels and types of nurse staffing in hospitals have been linked with mortality rates, medication errors, wound infections, hospital lengths of stay, urinary tract infections, and pneumonia (Clarke 2007). Based on such studies, in 2004, the importance of nurse staffing to hospital patient outcomes was recognized by the National Quality Forum (2004) in its published report, *National Voluntary Consensus Standards for Nursing-Sensitive Care: An Initial Performance Measure Set.* More recently, the CMS (2011b) has added "participation in a systematic clinical database registry for nursing sensitive care" to its Hospital Inpatient Quality Reporting Program (formerly known as Reporting Hospital Quality Data for Annual Payment Update Program), further emphasizing the critical link between nurse staffing and quality.

Consider the impact of human resources on the financial resources of an organization. Employee turnover can be costly. Filling a vacant position for a registered nurse can cost an acute care hospital from $82,000 to $88,000 (Jones 2008), and organizational turnover costs have been estimated between 3.4 percent and 5.8 percent of the annual operating budget at one large academic medical center (Waldman et al. 2010). In environments of scarce resources, expenses associated with preventable staff turnover may be viewed as quality waste within the managerial domain. McHugh and colleagues' (2010) *Using Workforce Practices to Drive Quality Improvement: A Guide for Hospitals* provides managers with a summary of best human resources practices.

Team Tools

Many required and recommended patient safety initiatives are accompanied by operational tools to promote teamwork. For example, The World Health Organization (WHO) Surgical Safety Checklist is shown in Exhibit 11.2. Built into this tool are recommendations for the specific team members required for the three verification steps.

Managers today may draw from a growing number of evidence-based tools that promote team effectiveness and enhance communication within and between teams to aid in institutionalizing desired team behaviors.

Summary

The importance of the manager's role in team design cannot be overestimated. Shared team expectations and role definitions along with defined

EXHIBIT 11.2
WHO Surgical
Safety Checklist

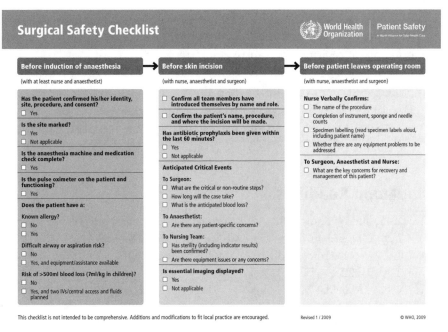

communication processes are necessary to promote effective teamwork and prevent breakdowns. Mental models about authority, hierarchy, talents, and differences in the workplace can influence the design and execution of teamwork. Managers should examine their mental models and incorporate an understanding of mental models that define the context of the work environment and design the structure in which teams operate.

Exercise

Background: The three principles of total quality—customer focus, continuous improvement, and teamwork—were introduced in Chapter 1. The objective of Chapter 7's exercise is to practice identifying management behaviors that demonstrate a focus on customers. This exercise uses the same case study to focus on the other two principles of total quality.

Objectives:
The objectives of this exercise are to:

- Practice identifying management behaviors that demonstrate teamwork and continuous improvement.
- Explore how teamwork and continuous improvement influence the patient experience.

Instructions:
- Read the case study at the end of Chapter 7.
- Describe several examples of how management demonstrated the principle of continuous improvement in the case study.
- Describe several examples of how management demonstrated the principle of teamwork in the case study.
- Describe how your responses to the two previous instructions contributed to the quality of the patient's experience (service quality) and the quality of the clinical service (content quality).

Companion Readings

Kelly, D. L., and N. Short. 2006. "Exploring Assumptions About Teams." *The Joint Commission Journal on Quality and Patient Safety* 32 (2): 109–12.

Rubin, I. 1996. "Learning How to Learn: The Key to CQI." *Physician Executive* 22 (10): 22–27.

Salas E., S. A. Almeida, M. Salisbury, H. King, E. H. Lazzara, R. Lyons, K. A. Wilson, P. A. Almeida, and R. McQuillan. 2009. "What Are the Critical Success Factors for Team Training in Health Care?" *The Joint Commission Journal on Quality and Patient Safety* 35 (8): 398–405.

Web Resources

AHRQ TeamSTEPPS Program: http://teamstepps.ahrq.gov/

Clinical Microsystems: http://clinicalmicrosystem.org/

Josie King Foundation: http://josieking.org

Veterans Administration National Center on Patient Safety: www.patientsafety.gov

World Health Organization, *Learning from Error*, Chapter 6, "Communication and Effective Team Working Between Health Care Workers." [Video] www.who.int/patientsafety/education/vincristine_download/en/index.html

Frameworks About Talents and Differences

The Meyers-Briggs Foundation: www.myersbriggs.org/my-mbti-personality-type/mbti-basics/

StrengthsFinder: http://strengths.gallup.com/110659/Homepage.aspx

Keirsey.com: http://keirsey.com/default.aspx

Human Dynamics International: www.humandynamics.com/

PRACTICE LAB

When asked how to get to Carnegie Hall, a famous musician replied, "Practice, practice, practice!"

The Section I end-of-chapter exercises are designed to aid students in remembering and understanding systems concepts. The Section II end-of-chapter exercises are designed to promote the understanding and application of the content. Section III includes additional exercises and case studies designed for students to further apply, evaluate, and synthesize the content and to individualize application to their own practice setting.

EXERCISE 1: REFLECTIVE JOURNAL

Although reflection plays an important role in personal learning, it is not practiced often in today's demanding work environments. To individualize the learning and enhance the relevance of the content, this journal assignment is offered as a teaching tool to tailor the content to the reader's practice environment, professional experience, and learning needs. This journal exercise section provides a structured opportunity for reflection on how the concepts discussed and the readings recommended in this book can be applied to circumstances and challenges in the work setting.

The journal may be used to reflect on an individual chapter or article or to synthesize content from a group of assigned readings that comprise a lesson or module.

Part I: Key Points to Remember

Depending on a reader's experience and current circumstances, one topic may be particularly relevant to one reader, but the same concept may be repetitive or routine to another reader. This question asks readers what lessons are important to them rather than instructing readers to consider someone else's perspective.

Part II: New Questions

Asking readers to list the questions that arise as a result of the readings emphasizes the importance of posing questions and helps develop critical thinking. Although readers, particularly students, may be accustomed to striving for the correct answers, this part of the journal is intended to encourage the practice of formulating good questions.

Part III: Application

Part III encourages readers to think about how the content may be applied to their own work environment or professional practice. Sometimes the content is relevant personally; a personal application is appropriate to include. The key is to be specific and concrete to solidify the understanding of the material and its practical uses.

Suggested Format for Reflective Journal

Name:

Date:

Citation(s):

I. Key points to remember from this reading and my reason(s) for selecting these points:

II. This information has prompted the following questions:

III. How I can use the information in my professional practice, in my work setting, or for my own personal effectiveness:

EXERCISE 2: THE MANAGER'S ROLE

Objective

To explore how managers influence the quality of products, services, and the customer experience.

Instructions

1. Think of an experience where you received or observed excellent quality. You may have had this experience as a customer, as a patient, as a provider, or as an employee. Describe the factors that made this an excellent experience and how you felt as a result of this experience. Using the list of management functions listed in Chapter 1 as a guide, include a description of management's influence on your experience. Do the same for a situation in which you experienced poor quality. Record your responses in the table or on one similar to it.

	Briefly describe the experience.	Describe what made this an excellent or poor quality experience.	How did you feel as a result?	What was manage-ment's role or influence?
Excellent quality experience				
Poor quality experience				

2. On the basis of the observations you recorded in the table, describe why it is important for health services managers to understand quality.

EXERCISE 3: DYNAMIC COMPLEXITY

Objective

To practice identifying dynamic complexity in a patient care experience.

Instructions

1. Read the case study.

2. Review the system characteristics that contribute to dynamic complexity:
    *   Change
    *   Trade-offs
    *   History dependency
    *   Tight coupling
    *   Nonlinearity

    For further explanation on these system characteristics, please refer to:

    Sterman, J. D. 2006. "Learning from Evidence in a Complex World."
    American Journal of Public Health 96 (3): 505–14.

3. Explain how these system characteristics are expressed in the case study on the following page.

Case Study

This case is adapted from Kelly, D. L., and S. L. Pestotnik. 1998. "Using Causal Loop Diagrams to Facilitate Double Loop Learning in the Healthcare Delivery Setting." Unpublished manuscript.

Mrs. B was a 66-year-old widow living on a fixed income. She had been diagnosed with high blood pressure and osteoporosis. Her private doctor knew her well. When he selected the medication with which to treat her high blood pressure, he took into account her age, the fact that she had osteoporosis, and other issues. He chose a drug that had proven beneficial for patients like Mrs. B and that had minimum side effects. Mrs. B did well on the medication for ten years. Her insurance covered the cost of her medication, except for a small out-of-pocket copayment.

The last time Mrs. B went to her local pharmacy to refill her prescription, the pharmacist informed her that her insurance company had contracted with a pharmacy benefits management (PBM) company. (The role of a PBM company is to perform a variety of cost-cutting services for health insurance plans. One of these services is to decide which drugs an insurance company will pay for; the PBM company's preferred-product list is known as a formulary.) If Mrs. B wanted to continue to take the same medication, it would cost her five times her usual copayment. She was quite disturbed because she could not afford this price increase and did not fully understand her insurance company's new policy. The pharmacist offered to call Mrs. B's doctor, explain the situation, and ask him whether he would change her prescription to the PBM-preferred brand. When the physician was contacted, he was not aware of the PBM company's action and was not completely familiar with the preferred product. The pharmacist discussed Mrs. B's predicament with the physician and described the financial consequences of her continuing to receive her original prescription. After this discussion with the pharmacist, the physician concluded that his only option was to approve the switch, which he did.

Mrs. B began taking the new brand of high-blood-pressure medicine. One week after starting on the new drug, she developed a persistent cough that aggravated her osteoporosis and caused her rib pain. When the cough and pain continued for another week, Mrs. B began to take over-the-counter medicines for the pain. She unknowingly opened herself to a reaction between her blood pressure medication and the pain medication: orthostatic hypotension (lightheadedness when rising from a lying to an upright position). One morning on her way to the bathroom, she fainted, fell, and broke her hip. She was admitted to the hospital for surgery, where she developed a urinary tract infection. The infection spread to her repaired hip, which resulted in a bloodstream infection that eventually led to her death.

EXERCISE 4: MENTAL MODELS

Objective

To practice identifying how mental models or assumptions influence behavior in organizations.

Instructions

1. See the Mental Models Worksheet at the end of this exercise. An example of a mental model associated with the "fighting fires" management style in the context of a health services organization is followed by actions associated with that mental model. Next, an alternative (different, opposite) mental model for this type of management style is offered, followed by associated actions.

2. Choose the mental model that currently influences you or that you would like to influence your management approach and style. Circle that mental model on the worksheet.

3. Think of a mental model about the topic of "power and authority" in organizations. Describe your actions as a health services manager if your behavior was driven by this mental model. Think of an alternative mental model about "power and authority" in organizations. Describe your actions as a health services manager if your behavior was driven by this mental model. Write your response in the respective boxes on the worksheet.

4. Choose the mental model that currently influences you or that you would like to influence your management approach and style. Circle that mental model on the worksheet.

5. Repeat 3 and 4 for two topics of your own choice.

Mental Models Worksheet

Topic	Mental Model	Actions	Alternative Mental Model	Actions
"Fighting fires" management style	Putting out "fires" at work makes me feel important—like I have really accomplished something today.	Look for fires. Act in a reactive, rather than proactive, manner. Manage day to day rather than strategically. Encourage employees to depend on the manager to solve problems.	If I am constantly putting out fires, some work or management processes are not working well.	Prevent problems rather than react to problems in the workplace. Improve work processes rather than continually treat symptoms of process breakdowns. Encourage employees to solve problems and participate in improvement efforts.
Power and authority				
(Select a topic)				
(Select a topic)				

EXERCISE 5: SYSTEM RELATIONSHIPS

Objective

To practice identifying relationships within systems.

Instructions

1. This exercise builds on Exercise 2: The Manager's Role. To begin, review your responses to that exercise.

2. Review the four systems models presented in Chapter 4:
   - Three core process model
   - Healthcare Criteria for Performance Excellence System Framework
   - Systems model of organizational accidents
   - Socioecological framework

3. Choose the model you can best relate to at this time.

4. Look at both your excellent quality experience and your poor quality experience, paying particular attention to how you described the manager's role or influence. Transfer what you wrote about the manager's role/influence to the Systems Model Worksheet.

5. Now, think about those experiences from the perspective of the systems model you chose in question 3. Describe any additional insights gained about this experience by viewing it within the context of the systems perspective represented by the model. Write your responses in the Systems Model Worksheet.

Systems Model Worksheet

	Manager's role/influence	Additional understanding by viewing through systems perspective
Excellent quality experience		
Poor quality experience		

EXERCISE 6: SYSTEMS ERROR CASE STUDY AND ANALYSIS

Objective

To better understand Reason's Model of Organizational Accidents by identifying different types of errors and interventions to prevent them from becoming an actual sentinel event.

Instructions

1. Read the article by Katherine Eban, "Your Hospital's Deadly Secret," available at:
    http://katherineeban.com/2008/03/01/your-hospitals-deadly-secret-conde-nast-portfolio/.

2. Based on the information provided in the article, identify specific actions or decisions that proved to be errors at the different levels of the system. Write your responses in the first column of the worksheet that follows. Complete this column before moving on to question 3.

3. Identify specific interventions that would have helped the organization monitor or prevent the failures identified in the first column from occurring. Write your response in the second column. Be very specific and concrete in your responses.

4. Refer to Chapter 4 and the Chapter 4 companion readings to assist you in completing this exercise.

Organizational Errors Worksheet

Latent failures in the healthcare system level external to the hospital and its parent company	Leadership intervention to monitor or prevent failure from occurring
Latent failures at the level of the organization's leadership	Leadership intervention to monitor or prevent failure from occurring
Latent failures at the level of frontline management	Leadership intervention to monitor or prevent failure from occurring
Workplace preconditions surrounding this event	Leadership intervention to monitor or prevent failure from occurring
Active errors associated with this event	Leadership intervention to monitor or prevent failure from occurring

EXERCISE 7: CUSTOMER REQUIREMENTS

Objective

To encourage practicing managers or care providers to evaluate how they incorporate customer, client, and stakeholder requirements into their practice.

Instructions

1. Write a brief description of your organizational setting on the Customers Worksheet at the end of this exercise. This setting may be a practice, department, or program.

2. Identify your customers, clients, and/or stakeholders, and write them in the first column of the Customers Worksheet.

3. Complete the remaining columns of the worksheet for each customer, client, and stakeholder listed in the first column.

Customers Worksheet

Organizational Setting:

Customer/ client/ stakeholder	Expectation/ requirement	How do I know this?	What I do to meet that expectation/ requirement	How I know how well I meet that expectation/ requirement

Adapted from: Kelly, D. L. 2009. NURS 6772: "Quality Improvement and Data Analysis," University of Utah College of Nursing classroom discussion, 8/28/09.

EXERCISE 8: IMPROVEMENT CASE STUDY

Objective

To practice quality improvement tools by applying them to an improvement effort in an ambulatory care setting.

Instructions

1. Read the following case study.

2. Follow the instructions at the end of the case.

Case Study

Background

You have just been brought in to manage a portfolio of several specialty clinics in a large multi-physician group practice in an academic medical center. The clinics reside in a multi-clinic facility that houses primary care and specialty practices as well as a satellite laboratory and radiology and pharmacy services. The practice provides the following centralized services for each of its clinics: registration, payer interface (e.g., authorization), and billing. The CEO of the practice has asked you to initially devote your attention to Clinic X to improve its efficiency and patient satisfaction.

Access Process

A primary care physician (or member of the office staff), patient, or family member calls the receptionist at Clinic X to request an appointment. If the receptionist is in the middle of helping a patient in person, the caller is asked to hold. The receptionist then asks the caller, "How may I help you?" If the caller is requesting an appointment within the next month, the appointment date and time is made and given verbally to the caller. If the caller asks additional questions, the receptionist provides answers. The caller is then given the toll-free preregistration phone number and asked to preregister before the date of the scheduled appointment. If the requested appointment is beyond a 30-day period, the caller's name and address are put in a "future file" because physician availability is given only one month in advance. Every month, the receptionist reviews the future file and schedules an appointment for each person on the list, and a confirmation is automatically mailed to the caller.

When a patient preregisters, the financial office is automatically notified and performs the necessary insurance checks and authorizations for the appropriate insurance plan. If the patient does not preregister, when the patient arrives in the clinic on the day of the appointment and checks in with the specialty clinic receptionist, she is asked to first go to the central registration area to register. Any obvious problems with authorization are corrected before the patient returns to the specialty clinic waiting room.

Receptionist's Point of View

The receptionist has determined that the best way to not inconvenience the caller is to keep her on the phone for as short an amount of time as possible. The receptionist also expresses frustration with the fact that there are too many things to do at once.

Physician's Point of View

The physician thinks too much of his time is spent on paperwork and chasing down authorizations. The physician senses that appointments are always running behind and that patients are frustrated, no matter how nice he is to them.

Patient's Point of View

Patients are frustrated when asked to wait in a long line to register, which makes them late for their appointments, and when future appointments are scheduled without their input. As a result of this latter factor, and work or childcare conflicts, patients often do not show up for these scheduled appointments.

Office Nurse's Point of View

The office nurse feels that he is playing catch up all day long and explaining delays. The office nurse also wishes there was more time for teaching.

Billing Office's Point of View

The billing office thinks some care is given that is not reimbursed because of inaccurate or incomplete insurance or demographic information or that care is denied authorization after the fact.

Data

On the Picker Institute website (pickerinstitute.org), you find the following patient expectations and dimensions of care for adults and children in their outpatient experiences with a hospital or clinic outpatient appointment:

- Respect for patients' values, preferences, and expressed needs
- Coordination and integration of care
- Information and education
- Physical comfort
- Emotional support and alleviation of fear and anxiety
- Involvement of family and friends
- Transition and continuity
- Access to care

Your last quarter's worth of performance data for the clinic is:

Overall satisfaction with visit	82%
Staff is courteous and helpful	90%
Waiting room time is less than 15 minutes	64%
Examination room waiting time is less than 15 minutes	63%
Patient no-show rate	20%
Patient cancellation rate	11%
Provider cancellation rate	10%
Preregistration rate	16%
Average number of patient visits per day	16
Range of patient visits per day	10–23

Instructions

1. Completely read all of the instructions.

2. Decide which problem you want to focus on as your first priority. Describe the problem and why you chose this problem.

3. State the goal for the improvement effort.

4. Identify the fundamental knowledge that is required on the team to solve this problem. Define the people you will invite to participate on the team and the fundamental knowledge they bring to the team.

5. Document the current process (as it is described in the case narrative) using a process flowchart.

6. Identify your customers and their expectations.

7. Explore and prioritize root causes of the problem by doing the following:

   a. Brainstorm root causes and document the causes on a fishbone diagram.

   b. Describe how you would collect data about how frequently the root causes contribute to the problem.

   c. Generate hypothetical data for question 7b. Make a Pareto chart using the hypothetical data for question 7b.

8. Review the following change concepts (Langley et al. 1996). Select and explain the ones that apply to improving your process. Be sure to take into account what you have learned in steps 5 through 7.

   a. Eliminate waste (e.g., things that are not used, intermediaries, unnecessary duplication)

   b. Improve workflow (e.g., minimize handoffs, move steps in the process closer together, find and remove bottlenecks, do tasks in parallel, adjust to high and low volumes)

   c. Manage time (e.g., reduce set-up time and waiting time)

   d. Manage variation (create standard processes where appropriate)

   e. Design systems to avoid mistakes (use reminders)

9. Incorporating what you learned in steps 5 through 8, improve the process and document the improved process with a process flowchart or workflow diagram.

10. Decide what you will measure to monitor the voice of the process and briefly describe how you would collect the data.

11. You have completed the "Plan" phase of the Shewhart cycle. Describe briefly how you would complete the rest of the PDCA cycle.

12. Save your answers to each part of this exercise. This will become the documentation of your improvement effort.

EXERCISE 9: TEAM GUIDELINES

Objective

To practice establishing team guidelines that capitalize on the strengths of team members.

Background

Often, team guidelines suggest rules of behavior such as "we will start on time" or "do not interrupt while another person is talking." This exercise offers an alternative approach to establishing team guidelines that enhances the team's ability to use team member strengths, increases the team's effectiveness, and improves the quality of the team's output.

Instructions

1. Define roles in your group. These roles may stay the same or may rotate among team members to provide an opportunity for each team member to practice each role.

2. Select and agree on group rules. These rules represent guidelines and expectations for how individuals and the group will function to promote the accomplishment of the team's assignment. As a start, the following rules are suggested. Add group rules as desired.
   - Give your full attention.
   - Be respectful of others.
   - Accept responsibility for the team's success.

3. Identify and discuss each team member's strengths and limitations. Record these characteristics on the following worksheet. Use this worksheet as a reference for your team.

Team Member Strengths Worksheet

Name	My unique contribution to this project team (e.g., experience, education, perspective, skill, background)	What I am least effective at doing (it is not that I am unwilling to try, it is just not my strength)

EXERCISE 10: GENERATIONAL DIFFERENCES

Objective

To explore the influence of generational differences on teams and teamwork in the health services setting

Background

The approach to understanding talents and differences among team members in the workplace presented is only one of many ways that diversity is represented in health services organizations. Another contributor to diverse perspectives is generational differences.

Instructions

1. Read: Olson, V. D. 2008. "Generational Diversity: Implications for Healthcare Leaders." *Journal of Business & Economics Research* 6 (11): 27–31.

2. If you work in a clinical setting, write a brief response to the question: How might an awareness of generational differences contribute to quality and safe patient care in my practice setting?

3. If you work in a non-clinical setting, write a brief response to the question: How might an awareness of generational differences contribute to effective teamwork and quality results in my work setting?

EXERCISE 11: ORGANIZATIONAL SELF-ASSESSMENT

Objectives

- To practice using an organizational assessment as a means of documenting current reality and identifying performance gaps
- To practice using the Baldrige Performance Excellence Program Health Care Criteria for Performance Excellence as a guide for completing an organizational assessment
- To conduct a "mini-assessment" of your organization

Note: Working managers may complete this exercise based on the practices of their own organizations. Students may complete this exercise based on the practices of a current or previous employer.

Instructions

1. Select and describe the boundaries of the system of interest; the term "organization" will be used to refer to this selected system. You may select a team, a department, a small organization (e.g., an office practice), or an entire organization.
2. To familiarize yourself with the criteria, review the section called "Category and Item Descriptions" in the Baldrige Criteria for Performance Excellence available from: www.nist.gov/baldrige/publications/hc_criteria.cfm
3. The Organizational Assessment Worksheet provides a general description of the criteria category followed by selected questions from the respective 2011–2012 Health Care Criteria for Performance Excellence category.
4. Based on the system selected in question 1, write a brief reply to the selected questions.

Organizational Assessment Worksheet

(taken from the 2011–2012 Health Care Criteria for Performance Excellence)

Organizational Profile (pp. 4, 6)

This category is a snapshot of your organization, including the key influences that affect how it operates and the key challenges it faces.

Briefly describe your organization, including its services; size; geographic community; key patient or customer groups; and current facilities, equipment, and technology, as well as the number of patients or clients it serves.

Briefly describe your organization's key challenges and your organization's current performance improvement system.

Leadership (p. 7)

This category examines how your organization's senior leaders' personal actions guide and sustain your organization. Also examined are your organization's governance system and how your organization fulfills its legal, ethical, and societal responsibilities and supports its key communities.

How do senior leaders deploy your organization's vision and values through your leadership system, to the workforce, to key suppliers and partners, and to patients and stakeholders as appropriate?

How do senior leaders encourage frank two-way communication throughout the organization?

Strategic Planning (pp. 10, 11)

This category examines how your organization develops strategic objectives and action plans. Also examined are how your chosen strategic objectives and action plans are deployed and changed, if circumstances require, and how progress is measured.

How does your organization conduct strategic planning?

Summarize your organization's action plans, how they are deployed, and key action plan performance measures or indicators.

Customer Focus (p. 13)

This category examines how your organization engages its patients and stakeholders for long-term marketplace success. This engagement strategy includes how your organization listens to the voice of its customers (your patients and stakeholders), builds customer relationships, and uses customer information to improve and identify opportunities for innovation.

How do you identify patient, stakeholder, and market requirements for service offerings?

How do you build and manage relationships with patients and stakeholders to meet their requirements and exceed their expectations at each stage of their relationship with you?

Measurement, Analysis, and Knowledge Management (p. 16)

This category examines how your organization selects, gathers, analyzes, manages, and improves its data, information, and knowledge assets and how it manages its information technology. It also examines how your organization uses review findings to improve its performance.

What are your key organizational performance measures?

How do you use these data and information to support organizational decision making and innovation?

Workforce Focus (p. 18)

This category examines your ability to assess workforce capability and capacity needs and to build a workforce environment conducive to high performance. This category examines how your organization engages, manages, and develops your workforce to utilize its full potential in alignment with your organization's overall mission, strategy, and action plans.

How do you assess your workforce capability and capacity needs, including skills, competencies, and staffing levels?

How do you address workplace environmental factors to ensure and improve workplace health, safety, and security?

Operational Focus (pp. 21, 22)

This category examines how your organization designs, manages, and improves its work systems and work processes to deliver patient and stakeholder value and achieve organizational success and sustainability. Also examined is your readiness for emergencies.

How do you design and innovate your work processes to meet all the key requirements?

How do you improve your work processes to improve healthcare outcomes, to achieve better performance, to reduce variability, and to improve healthcare services?

Organizational Performance Results (pp. 23–25)

This category examines your organization's performance and improvement in all key areas: healthcare and process outcomes, customer-focused outcomes, workforce-focused outcomes, leadership and governance outcomes, and financial and market outcomes. Performance levels are examined relative to those of competitors and other organizations with similar healthcare service offerings.

Provide data for one key measure or indicator of healthcare outcomes that is important to your patients and stakeholders.

Provide data for one key measure or indicator of patient or stakeholder satisfaction.

Provide data for one key measure or indicator of financial performance.

Provide data for one key measure or indicator related to operational performance.

Provide data for one key measure related to achieving legal, regulatory, and accreditation requirements.

Prioritizing Improvement Opportunities

1. Review the responses to the organizational assessment questions.

2. Note any questions for which you could not provide a response (i.e., the organization does not have a defined process or approach to address the topic of the question).

3. Review the organizational performance results data.

4. Select one or more measures that demonstrate less than desirable results.

5. Select one item from question 2 or 4 as the performance gap for the performance improvement exercise (see Exercise 12).

EXERCISE 12: IMPROVING A PERFORMANCE GAP IN MY ORGANIZATION

Objectives

- To provide an opportunity for managers to synthesize the concepts by being involved in a performance improvement effort using the actual identified needs in their own organizations
- To practice improvement approaches in a safe and controlled setting

Note: Implementing the results of this exercise in your own organization is not required. However, the exercise requires you to think through and document all of the steps in the exercise as if you were actually conducting this effort in your organization.

Instructions

1. Describe the performance gap selected from your Organizational Assessment (Exercise 11). This should be an area within the scope of your defined business unit or responsibilities.

2. Briefly describe the process(es) and/or functions that make up this performance area.

3. List who you would invite to participate in your improvement effort and why you selected these people.

4. Select one of the systems models (see Chapter 4). Explain insights gained by considering the process(es) described in question 2 within the context of the system relationships illustrated by this model.

5. a. State and critique several possible goal statements for this improvement effort. Use the Goals Worksheet to organize your thinking.

   b. Based on your critique, select the goal you will use for the improvement effort.

Goals Worksheet

Goal Statement	Type of Goal	Pros	Cons

6. Practice the purpose principle by asking yourself the following questions:
   - What am I trying to accomplish?

   - What is the purpose of the process(es) identified in question 2?

- Have I further expanded the purpose? What is the purpose of my previous response?

- Have I further expanded the purpose? What is the purpose of my previous response? (Continue expanding the purpose, if needed.)

- What larger purpose may eliminate the need to achieve this smaller purpose altogether?

- What is the right purpose for me to be working on? (Describe how this purpose differs or does not differ from the original purpose.)

7. Review your selected goal from question 5. After completing the purpose questions in question 6, does this still seem to be an appropriate goal? If not, redefine the goal of your improvement effort.

8. Is the process(es) from question 2 still the appropriate process to improve? If not, describe the process you will improve.

9. Describe the customers of the process and their expectations or requirements.

10. Describe a performance measure for this process (i.e., voice of the process) and how the data are collected. This may be the original performance indicator from which you determined this performance gap.

11. Document the high-level steps of the process as it currently exists using a flowchart.

12. Practice identifying mental models.
    - Identify at least two mental models that may be interfering with achieving a higher level of performance from your process. What actions are associated with these mental models?

    - Describe an alternative mental model for each that could enhance the improvement of your process. What actions are associated with the alternative mental model?

13. Practice infusing a different way of thinking into your improvement process based on the types discussed in Chapter 11.
    - Identify someone in your organization who appears to think in a different way than you do. Using the descriptions in Chapter 11, explain what led you to choose this person.

    - Review with this person your progress so far on this exercise.

    - Ask for this person's perspective and critique. Describe how this perspective complemented or contradicted your own.

    - Describe how you will or will not incorporate this new perspective into your improvement process.

14. Identify and apply any additional continuous quality improvement tools (see Chapter 10) that may help you better understand how to improve your process. Show your work.

15. Describe your ideal vision for this process. To help create your vision, ask yourself the following questions:
    If your process was the best practice for the community,
    • What would your process contribute to the overall organizational performance/effectiveness?

    • What would patients and families who are receiving care as a result of your process, or who are influenced by your process, say about their experience with your organization?

    • What would employees involved in your process say about the process?

    • What would colleagues around the country who came to learn from your best practice say about your process?

16. Improve your process.
    • Determine if you are solving a problem associated with an existing process or creating a new process.

    • Review your original and/or revised improvement goal(s).

    • Review the purpose of your process.

    • Review your customers' expectations.

- Review the mental models you selected.

- Review what you learned from question 14.

- Redefine the starting and ending points of your process as needed to support the purpose.

- Based on the aforementioned information, document the ideal process that will achieve the purpose you described using a high-level flowchart.

- Check your process against the goal you set for your improvement effort.

17. Review the measure from question 10 that you selected as the voice of the process. Is this measure still the appropriate indicator/measure for your ideal process (i.e., measures the voice of the process)? If not, what would that indicator/measure be?

18. Review your goal and your purpose. Will the above indicator/measure(s) help you determine if you are working toward your goal and carrying out your purpose?

19. Describe any unintended consequences to any other area, department, process, or entity within or outside of your organization if you change your process. What indicator/measure(s) would help you to be on the alert for them?

20. Describe how the indicators/measures from questions 17 and 19 fit into a balanced set of performance measures for the department/organization.

21. For your defined indicator/measures, describe:
How would you collect the data?

How often would you report the data?

With whom and how you would share your data for review on a regular basis?

22. You have defined the purpose and described the ideal process. Determine the ideal structure to carry out this process—that is, by whom and how should the process be carried out to best achieve the purpose?

23. Describe an implementation plan that takes into consideration the concepts described in Chapter 9.

EXERCISE 13: IMPROVING A PERFORMANCE GAP: A CASE STUDY

Objectives

- To synthesize the concepts in the book by being involved in a performance improvement effort using a case study that presents real conflicts in organizations
- To practice performance improvement in a safe and controlled setting

Notes

1. This exercise is designed for five teams of students. Teams may elect to tackle one of the five performance gaps presented in the case study.
2. The case study that accompanies this exercise is not a business case study (i.e., a detailed description and account of the organization), rather, it presents enough organizational context for readers to apply the concepts and tools described in this book.

Instructions

Read the case study and answer the questions that follow. The questions do not require you to have all the answers, but they lead you to ask the right questions. If you think you need more content information on certain areas (i.e., details about the organization or data), identify that need by defining the questions you would ask to obtain that information.

Case Study

Hospital Background

Last year, the hospital admitted 20,925 inpatients. For 1,000 of these total patient admissions, congestive heart failure (CHF) was documented as the primary or secondary diagnosis. Of these CHF patients, 48 percent were female and 52 percent were male, with a mean age of 63. Approximately 50 percent of these patients had a history of CHF, and approximately 50 percent were newly diagnosed. The average length of stay for a CHF patient with a primary or secondary diagnosis was 4.2 days. The payer mix for the group was 50 percent Medicare, 40 percent private payer, and 10 percent indigent or charity. As part of the hospital's three- to five-year plan to excel in cardiac services, the hospital has decided to focus on CHF as one of its goals this year.

Scenario One: Clinical Performance Gap

Your team represents internists and other clinical staff in an internal medicine practice.

Your interest in improving outcomes in patients with CHF prompted you to join a quality improvement project sponsored by your state quality improvement organization. As part of the project, your team helped clarify guidelines for this patient population in the areas of diagnosis, treatment, and self-management education. Each of the team members has been using these guidelines for the past year.

You have received the evaluation data for the project that show other hospitals' performance in the heart-failure indicators required by the Centers for Medicare & Medicaid Services. The report shows your hospital's overall performance, but you also receive individual reports showing how your CHF patients compare. Your performance is 10 to 20 percent better in each of the indicators compared with the performance of CHF patients in the hospital as a whole.

At the request of the hospital's medical staff president, you give a report on the quality improvement project at the next medical staff meeting. Of the 1,000 CHF patients typically admitted each year, your patients represent only one-tenth, but they demonstrate the best outcomes. As a result, the medical staff president asks your team to lead an effort to improve care to all patients admitted to the hospital with a primary or secondary diagnosis of CHF.

Scenario Two: Operational Performance Gap

Your team collectively represents the manager of the social work department at the hospital.

At the monthly staff meeting, you ask for input on the increasing number of overtime hours that you have observed on the payroll reports. The staff describes their frustrations with how discharge planning is done at the hospital. With shorter hospital stays, they are finding that they have more to do in less time. Responsibilities such as arranging transportation, ensuring that follow-up appointments have been scheduled, and arranging home and long-term care are becoming more difficult to accomplish.

Patients who are admitted for CHF and spend a day or two in the intensive care unit pose a particular problem. Many times, the social workers are not notified until the day the patient is supposed to be going home. As a result, everything becomes an emergency, which makes it hard for the social workers to manage their time effectively. You tell your staff that you will initiate an improvement effort on the discharge process and that you will begin with patients with CHF.

Scenario Three: Operational Performance Gap

Your team represents the nursing shift supervisors of the hospital.

A nursing supervisor is assigned to each shift and has the responsibility for clinical and administrative oversight of the nursing staff for that shift. Your specific responsibilities include monitoring and ensuring adequate nursing staff coverage on each shift; serving as a resource to unit charge nurses; assisting with emergencies, such as codes; serving as the administrative liaison for patient complaints that are out of the ordinary or that unit staff are unable to handle; ensuring that admissions, transfers, and discharges of patients between units or departments occur smoothly; and helping to resolve interdepartmental conflicts.

Recently, in an effort to cut costs, the hospital approved a proposal to eliminate the day-shift nursing supervisor. The rationale was that patient care unit managers (some of whom are traditional nurse managers and some of whom are nonclinical administrative managers) are present during the day and should be able to absorb the functions of the shift supervisor. Since this change was implemented, it has become more difficult for you and the other nursing supervisors to do your jobs on the evening and night shifts. One problem is that patients who should have been discharged in the morning are being delayed until the afternoon. Because your bed occupancy is typically around 80 percent, these delays are causing bottlenecks for new admissions from surgery and from the emergency department. In particular, the general medicine floors—including the telemetry unit where the CHF patients are and where approximately 70 percent of the admissions come through the emergency department—are faced with these problems. You have heard the following comments from nurses throughout the hospital:

- "The managers always seem to be at meetings and are never available, so it's like not having a supervisor on day shift."
- "When I take patients downstairs to the lobby to go home, I have always stopped at the outpatient pharmacy to get their prescriptions filled. Lately, I have had to wait in line for 45 minutes!"
- "The doctors won't discharge patients until they see the morning blood work results. Since the lab work isn't drawn until 8:00 am, by the time I get the results back and track down the doctor to get the OK for discharge, it's usually close to noon."

Scenario Four: Administrative Performance Gap

Your team collectively represents the administrator for the cardiac service line.

The following departments report to you: the medicine/telemetry unit, the coronary care unit, the thoracic intensive care unit (i.e., heart surgery unit), the cardiac rehabilitation unit, the cardiac catheterization laboratory, and the electrocardiogram and echocardiogram laboratories. You are also the administrative liaison to the cardiologists and thoracic surgeons.

Because the nursing department is decentralized, you have a nursing director who is dedicated to your service line. She has just left your office after describing the complaints she has been receiving from the emergency department: patients are backing up in the emergency department as a result of delays in admitting patients to the general medicine floors, particularly the telemetry unit. The emergency department reports to the administrator responsible for the trauma service line.

You have just been recruited from out of state and are new to this position. You were hired with the expectation that you would improve the coordination of care for patients in your service line. The managers who report to you get together monthly for a managers' meeting. So far you have learned that these meetings have not been very useful in assisting managers with the issues that they consider important. Your predecessor had a traditional command-and-control style, and the managers feel stifled when trying to make the improvements they want to make in their respective departments. You want to help your managers be more effective both individually and as a team.

Scenario Five: Leadership Performance Gap

Your team represents the CEO of the hospital.

You have been in the position for ten years, and your previous position was as a senior administrator. In the past few years, your job has become much more difficult: patients are sicker, lengths of stay are shorter, compliance and other regulations keep accumulating, staff turnover is increasing, and workforce shortages are more prevalent. Every time you go to a professional meeting, you hear of another colleague who has been "reorganized" out of a job. You feel fortunate to have remained in your position for so long, but at its last meeting, the board made it clear that the hospital's quality must improve. Your responsibility is to ensure that the board's requests are carried out. At first this expectation seems unreasonable, given that so many things in the industry are not under your control.

Since returning from an executive leadership conference a few weeks ago, you have been doing a lot of soul searching. Your management approach has always worked in the past, but it does not seem to be working anymore. You were intrigued by one of the keynote speakers at the conference, who described the attributes required by healthcare leaders today. The speaker said that "a good leader is one whom others trust and have confidence in following because of that leader's values, vision, capabilities, and expertise in handling unstable and difficult situations"; management of frustration, anxiety, and conflict is particularly admired. Such a leader keeps "human suffering as the uppermost concern" and enables groups to "effectively manage surprises." A truly good leader is "able to identify and help guide innovative projects through various forums—strategic, scientific, economic/business, or political . . . the type of leader required in healthcare today has detailed knowledge of a variety of disciplines that are required to make a healthcare organization work well and has an insatiable curiosity to learn those disciplines that are unfamiliar" (Pierce 2000, 25–26).

You decide that, starting today, you will reinvent yourself in an effort to meet the board's expectations.

Case Study Questions

1. Select the performance gap that you will improve. In a few sentences, describe the performance gap.

2. Briefly describe the process(es) and/or functions that make up this performance area.

3. List who you would invite to participate in your improvement effort and why you selected these people.

4. Select one of the systems models (see Chapter 4). Explain insights gained by considering the process(es) described in question 2 within the context of the system relationships illustrated by this model.

5. a. State and critique several possible goal statements for the improvement effort. Use the Goals Worksheet to organize your thinking.

   b. Based on your critique, select the goal you will use for the improvement effort.

Goals Worksheet

Goal Statement	Type of Goal	Pros	Cons

6. Practice the purpose principle by asking yourself the following questions:

- What am I trying to accomplish?

- What is the purpose of the process(es) identified in question 2?

- Have I further expanded the purpose? What is the purpose of my previous response?

- Have I further expanded the purpose? What is the purpose of my previous response? (Continue expanding the purpose, if needed.)

- What larger purpose may eliminate the need to achieve this smaller purpose altogether?

- What is the right purpose for me to be working on? (Describe how this purpose differs or does not differ from the original purpose.)

7. Review your selected goal from question 5. After completing the purpose questions in question 6, does this still seem to be an appropriate goal? If not, redefine the goal of your improvement effort.

8. Is the process(es) from question 2 still the appropriate process to improve? If not, describe the process you will improve.

9. Describe the customers of the process and their expectations or requirements.

10. Describe a performance measure for this process (i.e., voice of the process) and how the data are collected.

11. Document the high-level steps of the process as it currently exists using a flowchart.

12. Practice identifying mental models.
    - Identify at least two mental models that may be interfering with achieving a higher level of performance from your process. What actions are associated with these mental models?

    - Describe an alternative mental model for each that could enhance the improvement of your process. What actions are associated with the alternative mental models?

13. Identify and apply any additional continuous quality improvement tools (see Chapter 10) that may help you better understand how to improve your process. Show your work.

14. Describe your ideal vision for this process. To help create your vision, you may ask yourself the following questions.

    If your process was the best practice for the community,

    • What would your process contribute to the overall organizational performance and effectiveness?

    • What would patients and families who are receiving care as a result of your process, or who are influenced by your process, say about their experience with your organization?

    • What would employees involved in your process say about the process?

    • What would colleagues around the country who came to learn from your best practice say about your process?

15. Improve your process.

    • Determine if you are solving a problem associated with an existing process or creating a new process.

    • Review your original and/or revised improvement goal(s).

    • Review the purpose of your process.

    • Review your customers' expectations.

    • Review the mental models you selected.

- Review what you learned from question 13.

- Redefine the starting and ending points of your process as needed to support the purpose.

- Based on the aforementioned information, document the ideal process that will achieve the purpose you described using a high-level flowchart.

- Check your process against the goal you set for your improvement effort.

16. Review the measure from question 10 that you selected as the voice of the process. Is this measure still appropriate for your ideal process? If not, what would that measure be?

17. Review your goal and your purpose. Would the above measure(s) help you determine if you are working toward your goal and carrying out your purpose?

18. Describe any unintended consequences to any other area, department, process, or entity within or outside of your organization if you change your process. What indicators/measures would help you to be on the alert for them?

19. Describe how the indicators/measures from questions 16 and 18 fit into a balanced set of performance measures for the department or organization.

20. For your defined indicators/measures, describe the following:
    - How would you collect the data?

    - How often would you report the data?

    - With whom and how would you share your data for review on a regular basis?

21. You have defined the purpose and described the ideal process. Determine the ideal structure to carry out this process—that is, by whom and how should the process be carried out to best achieve the purpose?

22. Describe an implementation plan that takes into consideration the concepts described in Chapter 9.

GLOSSARY OF TERMS

Accountable care organization (ACO): an organization through which groups of providers share responsibility for providing care (Gold 2011)

Accreditation: a form of external quality review for health services organizations based on defining quality standards, assessing organizational compliance, and recognizing compliant organizations (Rooney and Ostenburg 1999)

Active errors: errors committed by frontline workers; the results are seen immediately (Reason 1990, 1997)

Adverse event: "an injury caused by medical management rather than the underlying condition of the patient" (IOM 1999, 4)

Allocative policies: policies "designed to provide net benefits to some distinct group or class of individuals or organizations, at the expense of others, to ensure that public objectives are met" (Longest 2010, 13)

Assignable variation: also referred to as special cause variation resulting from something irregular (i.e., not inherent to the process) (Carey and Lloyd 2001)

Attribute: also referred to as discrete data, "counts of events that can be aggregated into discrete categories" (Carey and Lloyd 2001, 70)

Balanced scorecard (BSC): a "set of measures that gives top managers a fast but comprehensive view of the business. The balanced scorecard includes financial measures that tell the results of actions already taken. And it complements the financial measures with operational measures on customer satisfaction, internal processes, and the organization's innovation and improvement activities—operational measures that are the drivers of future financial performance" (Kaplan and Norton 2005, 174)

Cause-and-effect diagram: (also referred to as a fishbone or Ishikawa diagram) is a tool for organizing and documenting causes of a problem in a structured format

Certification: a form of external quality review for health services professionals and organizations; when applied to individuals, it represents advanced education and competence; when applied to organizations, it represents meeting predetermined standards for a specialized service provided by the organization (Rooney and Ostenburg 1999)

Cognitive psychology: the branch of psychology "concerned with all forms of cognition—the mental activities involved in acquiring and processing information—including attention, perception, learning, memory, thinking, problem solving, decision making and language"(*Dictionary of Psychology Online* 2009a)

Complex: the presence of a large number of variables that interact with each other in innumerable ways

Context (1): "the unquestioning assumptions through which all experience is filtered" (Davis 1982)

Context (2): "the interrelated conditions in which something exists or occurs" (Merriam-Webster Dictionary Online 2010a)

Creative tension: the discrepancy between an organization's current level of performance and its desired level and vision for the future

Crew resource management (CRM): team approach that accepts errors as inevitable and includes "a set of error countermeasures with three lines of defense. The first, naturally, is the avoidance of error. The second is trapping incipient errors before they are committed. The third and last is mitigating the consequences of those errors that occur and are not trapped" (Helmreich, Merritt, and Wilhelm 1999, 27)

Critical thinking: "the art of analyzing and evaluating thinking with a view to improving it" (Critical Thinking Community 2010)

Customer: user or potential user of one's services or programs

Delivery quality: also referred to as "service quality"; refers to the interpersonal components of care (e.g., empathy and communication) and to how well a patient's requirements and expectations are being met (e.g., access, timely billing)

Deployment flowchart: process flowchart diagram that includes and distinguishes who is responsible for which steps of the process

Double-loop learning: In double-loop learning, if one is not satisfied with the results or consequences, before taking action, underlying assumptions are examined, clarified, communicated, and/or reframed based on what the assumptions reveal. Only then is subsequent action, based on lessons revealed, taken (Argyris 1991; Tagg 2007)

Dynamic complexity: where "cause and effect are subtle, and where the effects over time of interventions are not obvious" (Senge 2006, 71)

Errors: "all those occasions in which a planned sequence of mental or physical activities fails to achieve its intended outcome" (Reason 1990, 9)

Error of commission: something that should not be done is done

Error of omission: something that should be done is not done

Execution error: proper plan carried out improperly

External customer: a user outside the organization

FMEA: failure mode and effects analysis; a systematic process used to conduct a prospective analysis

Goal: a desired end

Health policies: policies that "pertain to health or influence the pursuit of health" (Longest 2010, 6)

High-reliability organizations (HROs): "organizations with systems in place that are exceptionally consistent in accomplishing their goals and avoiding potentially catastrophic errors" (AHRQ 2008b)

Individual tracer: The Joint Commission's in-depth examination that follows a patient's experience within the organization

Internal customer: a user within the organization

The Joint Commission: a private accreditation body for numerous types of services organizations

Judgment errors: improper selection of an objective or a plan of action

Latent errors: errors occurring in the upper levels of the organization; the error may lie dormant for days or years until a particular combination of circumstances allows the latent error to become an adverse event (Reason 1990, 1997)

Lean thinking: an improvement philosophy based on eliminating waste

Licensure: granted by a governmental body and represents *minimum* standards

Mental model: a deeply ingrained way of thinking that influences how a person sees and understands the world as well as how that person acts

Microsystem (clinical): "a small group of people who work together on a regular basis to provide care to discrete subpopulations of patients . . . a microsystem is the local milieu in which patients, providers, support staff, information, and processes converge for the purpose of providing care to individual people to meet their health needs" (Nelson et al. 2007)

Mission: statement that defines the system's identity

Nonlinear: the "effect is rarely proportional to the cause" (Sterman 2000, 22)

Optimizing violations: "actions taken to further personal rather than task-related goals" (Reason 1995, 82)

Organization: "social structures created by individuals to support the collaborative pursuit of specified goals" (Scott 2003, 11)

Organizational design: "How the building blocks of the organization (authority, responsibility, accountability, information, and rewards) are arranged and rearranged to improve effectiveness and adaptive capacity" (Shortell and Kaluzny 2006, 316)

Organizational effectiveness: a theoretical base resulting from the overlap of quality and management schools of thought that helps managers to better understand and explain the organization (management theory) and also to improve the organization (total quality theory) (Dean and Bowen 2000)

Organizational structure: how responsibility and authority are distributed throughout an organization (Shortell and Kaluzny 2006)

Outcome: "a change in a patient's current and future health status that can be attributed to antecedent healthcare" (Donabedian 1980, 79, 81–83)

Pareto chart: bar graph that displays data in descending order (most important/ most frequent to least important/least frequent) and also displays cumulative totals using a line graph when reading from left to right

Pareto Principle: "most effects come from relatively few causes; that is, 80 percent of the effects come from 20 percent of the possible causes" (2011, 54).

Patient safety: "freedom from accidental or preventable injuries produced by medical care" (AHRQ 2010b).

Performance management: "an umbrella term that describes the methodologies, metrics, processes and systems used to monitor and manage the business performance of an enterprise" (Buytendijk and Rayner 2002).

Performance management cycle: links the performance standards, performance measurement, performance improvement, and reporting progress in an ongoing cycle

PEST: political, economic, social, technological analysis

Pharmacogenomics: "a science that examines the inherited variations in genes that dictate drug response and explores the ways these variations can be used to predict whether a patient will have a good response to a drug, a bad response to a drug, or no response at all" (NCBI 2004)

Pharmacotherapeutics: "the study of the therapeutic uses and effects of drugs" (Medline Plus Merriam-Webster Medical Dictionary 2011)

Policy: "a definite course or method of action selected from among alternatives and in light of given conditions to guide and determine present and future decisions" (Merriam-Webster Dictionary Online 2011)

Primary prevention: preventing a disease or disorder before it happens (Merrill and Timmreck 2006, 16)

Private sector policy: rules that guide governance and operations within a specific organization or as established by private organizations for the purpose of industry oversight (Longest 2010)

Process: an organized group of related activities that work together to transform one or more kinds of input into outputs that are of value to the customer (ASQ 2002)

Process flowchart: a picture of the sequence of steps in a process

Process of care: "a set of activities that go on within and between practitioners and patients" (Donabedian 1980, 79, 81–83)

Prospective analysis: a proactive, preventive approach to improvement that anticipates potential problems and improves processes in advance of a problem occurring

Public policy: "authoritative decisions made in the legislative, executive, or judicial branches of government that are intended to direct or influence the actions, behaviors, or decisions of others" (Longest 2010, 5)

Purpose: an identity or a reason for being

Purpose principle: a tool to aid managers in identifying the right purpose to address

Quality: "The degree to which health services for individuals and populations increase the likelihood of desired health outcomes and are consistent with current professional knowledge" (Lohr 1990, 21)

Quality assurance (QA): eliminating defective outputs

Quality control (QC): "the operational techniques and activities used to fulfill requirements for quality" (ASQ 2011)

Quality improvement (QI): improving defective processes to improve the quality of the outputs

Quality management: the manager's role and contribution to organizational effectiveness; how managers operating in various types of health services organizations and settings understand, explain, and continuously improve their organizations to allow them to deliver quality and safe patient care, promote quality patient and organizational outcomes, and improve health in their communities

Random variation: also referred to as common cause variation; the natural variation present in the process

Regulatory policy: policy used to promote societal objectives in situations in which private markets do not function properly according to competitive market rules (Longest 2010)

Repair service behavior: a type of problem solving where organizations or individuals solve a problem they know how to solve, whether or not it is the problem they need to solve (Dorner 1996)

Root cause analysis: "a process for identifying basic or causal factor(s) underlying variation in performance, including the occurrence or possible occurrence of a sentinel event" (Croteau 2010)

Routine violations: when a step in a process is intentionally skipped; cutting-corners activities

Run chart: a graphic representation of data over time where the x-axis represents the time interval and the y-axis represents the variable of interest

Schema: a "mental representation of some aspect of experience, based on prior experience and memory, structured in such a way as to facilitate (and sometimes to distort) perception, cognition, the drawing of inferences, or the interpretation of new information in terms of existing knowledge" (*Dictionary of Psychology Online* 2009b)

Secondary prevention: activities "aimed at health screening and detection activities [to] . . . block the progression of disease" (Merrill and Timmreck 2006, 17)

Sentinel event: "An unexpected occurrence involving death or serious physical or psychological injury, or the risk thereof. Serious injury specifically includes loss of limb or function. The phrase, 'or the risk thereof' includes any process variation for which a recurrence would carry a significant chance of a serious adverse outcome. Such events are called "sentinel" because they signal the need for immediate investigation and response (The Joint Commission 2010f)

Service quality: the "myriad characteristics that shape the experience of care for patients" (Kenagy, Berwick, and Shore 1999, 661) including interpersonal components of care (e.g., empathy and communication) and how well a patient's requirements and expectations are being met

Shewhart cycle: (also referred to as the PDCA cycle) consists of four continuous steps: plan, do, check/study, and act

Situation violations: occur when a person believes that the action "offer[s] the only path available to getting the job done and where the rules or procedures are seen as inappropriate for the present situation" (Reason 1995, 82)

Six Sigma: A rigorous and disciplined improvement approach using defined tools, methods, and statistical analysis with the goal of driving defects to zero

Six Sigma DMAIC: define, measure, analyze, improve, control

Small win: "a concrete, complete, implemented outcome of moderate importance" (Weick 1984, 43)

Stakeholder: "all groups that are or might be affected by an organization's services, actions or success" (NIST 2011, 63)

Structure: "the relatively stable characteristics of the providers of care, of the tools and resources they have at their disposal, and of the physical and organizational settings in which they work" (Donabedian 1980, 79, 81–83)

SWOT: strengths, weaknesses, opportunities, threats analysis

System: a collection of parts that interact with each other to form an interdependent whole (Kauffman 1980; Scott 2003)

Systemic structure: involves the interrelationships among key elements within the system and the influence of these interrelationships on the system's behavior over time (Senge 2006).

Systems thinking: "is a discipline for seeing wholes. It is a framework for seeing interrelationships, rather than things, for seeing patterns of change rather than static 'snap-shots' . . . and systems thinking is a sensibility—for the subtle interconnectedness that gives living systems their unique character" (Senge 2006, 68–69)

System tracer: The Joint Commission's in-depth examination of the multiple processes, systems, and structures that make up the priority areas such as infection control, medication management, data use, and environment of care

Team: a number of persons associated together in work or activity (Merriam-Webster Dictionary Online 2010c)

Technical quality: clinical expertise and technical aspects of healthcare

Tertiary prevention: intervention that "blocks the progression of a disability, condition, or disorder in order to keep it from advancing and requiring excessive care" (Merrill and Timmreck 2006, 17)

Tightly coupled: when the parts of a system "exhibit relatively time-dependent, invariant, and inflexible connections with little slack" (Scott 2003, 358)

Total quality (TQ): "a philosophy or an approach to management that can be characterized by its principles, practices, and techniques. Its three principles are customer focus, continuous improvement, and teamwork . . . each principle is implemented through a set of practices . . . the practices are, in turn, supported by a wide array of techniques (i.e., specific step-by-step methods intended to make the practices effective)" (Dean and Bowen 2000, 4–5).

Toyota Production System: Common method of applying Lean thinking in health services developed at the Toyota Motor Company

Tracer methodology: The Joint Commission's on-site survey method that provides the opportunity to examine the depth and breadth of an organization's quality and safety efforts

Value: ratio of quality to cost (value = quality / cost)

Variable: also referred to as continuous data; "take on different values on a continuous scale" (Carey and Lloyd 2001, 70)

Violations: deviations from safe operating practices, procedures, standards, or rules (Reason 1997, 72)

Vision: ideal future state

REFERENCES

Agency for Healthcare Research and Quality (AHRQ). 2011. CAHPS Survey Instruments. [Online information; retrieved 2/19/11.] www.cahps.ahrq .gov/content/products/Prod_Intro.asp?p=102&s=2

———. 2010a. Consumer Assessment of Healthcare Providers and Systems Program Website. [Online information; retrieved 8/23/10.] www.cahps.ahrq.gov

———. 2010b. "Patient Safety Network Glossary." [Online information; retrieved 6/21/10.] www.psnet.ahrq.gov/glossary.aspx

———. 2008a. *AHRQ Profile: Quality Research for Quality Healthcare.* AHRQ Publication No. 00-P005, August 2008. [Online information; retrieved 10/9/2010.] www.ahrq.gov/about/profile.htm

———. 2008b. *Becoming a High Reliability Organization: Operational Advice for Hospital Leaders.* AHRQ Publication No. 08-0022, Rockville, MD. [Online information; retrieved 8/31/10.] www.ahrq.gov/qual/hroadvice/

American Association of Colleges of Nursing. 2010. "Nursing Faculty Shortage Fact Sheet." [Online information; retrieved 6/22/10.] www.aacn.nche .edu/Media/FactSheets/FacultyShortage.htm

American Society for Quality (ASQ). 2011. "Glossary." [Online information; retrieved 3/9/11.] www.asq.org/glossary/index.html

———. 2010a. "ASQ The Global Voice of Quality." [Online information; retrieved 12/9/10.] http://asq.org/

———. 2010b. "Continuous Improvement." [Online article; retrieved 8/28/10.] www.asq.org/learn-about-quality/continuous-improvement/overview/ overview.html

———. 2010c. "Six Sigma." [Online article; retrieved 8/28/10.] www.asq.org/ learn-about-quality/six-sigma/overview/dmaic.html

———. 2010d. "Process View of Work." [Online article; retrieved 8/28/10.] www.asq.org/learn-about-quality/process-view-of-work/overview/ overview.html

———. 2002. "Quality Glossary." *Quality Progress* July: 43–61.

Apkon, M., J. Leonard, L. Probst, and R. Vitale. 2004. "Design of a Safer Approach to Intravenous Drug Infusions: Failure Mode Effects Analysis." *Quality and Safety in Healthcare* 13: 265–71.

Argyris, C. 1991. "Teaching Smart People How to Learn." *Harvard Business Review* 69 (3): 99–110.

Baars, I., S. Evers, A. Arnoud, and G. van Merod. 2009. "Performance Measurement in Mental Health Care: Present Situation and Future

Possibilites." *International Journal of Health Planning and Management* 25: 198–214.

Barquet, N., and P. Domingo. 1997. "Smallpox: The Triumph over the Most Terrible of the Ministers of Death." *Annals of Internal Medicine* 127: 635–42.

Benbow, D. W., and T. M. Kubiak. 2005. *The Certified Six Sigma Black Belt Handbook*. Milwaukee, WI: ASQ Quality Press.

Bingham, T. 2005. Unpublished document.

Blanton, G., T. B. Clapp, T. Nakajo, and C. S. Seastrunk. 2007. "Healthcare-Focused Error Proofing: Principles and Solution Directions for Reducing Human Errors." *ASQ Healthcare Update Newsletter* [Online article; retrieved 8/30/10.] http://asq.org/pdf/articles/healthcare-focused-error-proofing.pdf

Bond, C. A., C. L. Rachl, and T. Frank. 2002. "Clinical Pharmacy Services, Hospital Pharmacy Staffing, and Medication Errors in United States Hospitals." *Pharmacotherapy* 22: 134–47.

Burgmeier, J. 2002. "Failure Mode and Effect Analysis: An Application in Reducing Risk in Blood Transfusion." *The Joint Commission Journal on Quality Improvement* 28 (6): 331–39.

Buytendijk, F., and N. Rayner. 2002. "A Starter's Guide to CPM Methodologies." Research Note TU-16-2429. Stamford, CT: Gartner, Inc.

Caldwell, C. 2008. "Breakthrough Quality: What the Board Must Do." *Trustee* June: 32–33.

Carey, R. G., and R. C. Lloyd. 2001. *Measuring Quality Improvement in Healthcare: A Guide to Statistical Process Control Applications*. Milwaukee, WI: Quality Press.

Centers for Medicare & Medicaid Services (CMS). 2011a. "Hospital Compare." [Online article; retrieved 2/19/11.] www.hospitalcompare.hhs.gov

————. 2011b. "Reporting Hospital Quality Data for Annual Payment Update." [Online information; retrieved 1/13/2011.] www.cms.gov/HospitalQualityInits/08_HospitalRHQDAPU.asp

————. 2010a. "Conditions for Coverage & Conditions for Participation." [Online information; retrieved 10/15/2010.] www.cms.gov/CFCsAndCoPs/

————. 2010b. "HCAHPS: Patients' Perceptions of Care Survey." [Online information; retrieved 7/8/2010.] www.cms.gov/HospitalQualityInits/30_HospitalHCAHPS.asp

————. 2010c. "Hospital-Acquired Conditions (HAC) and Present on Admission (POA) Indicator Reporting Factsheet." [Online information; retrieved 10/16/2010.] www.cms.gov/HospitalAcqCond/downloads/HACFactsheet.pdf

————. 2010d. "Hospital Compare: Technical Appendix." [Online information; retrieved 10/16/2010.] www.hospitalcompare.hhs.gov/staticpages/for-professionals/poc/Technical-Appendix.aspx#POC3

————. 2010e. "Reporting Hospital Quality Data for Annual Payment Update." [Online information; retrieved 10/16/10.] www.cms.gov/HospitalQualityInits/08_HospitalRHQDAPU.asp

———. 2010f. "Roadmap for Implementing Value Driven Healthcare in the Traditional Medicare Fee-for-Service Program." [Online report; retrieved 10/16/2010.] www.cms.gov/QualityInitiativesGenInfo/downloads/VBPRoadmap_OEA_1-16_508.pdf.

———. 2010g. "Roadmap for Quality Measurement in the Traditional Medicare Fee-for-Service Program." [Online report; retrieved 6/25/10.] www.cms.gov/QualityInitiativesGenInfo/downloads/QualityMeasurementRoadmap_OEA1-16_508.pdf

Charmel, P. A. 2010. "Defining and Evaluating Excellence in Patient-Centered Care." *Frontiers of Health Services Management* 26 (4): 27–34.

Chassin, M. R., J. M. Loeb, S. P. Schmaltz, and R. M. Wachter. 2010. "Accountability Measures: Using Measurement to Promote Quality Improvement." *The New England Journal of Medicine* 363 (7): 683–88.

Clarke, S. P. 2007. "Nurse Staffing in Acute Care Settings: Research Perspectives and Practical Applications." *The Joint Commission Journal on Quality and Patient Safety* 33 (11s): 30–44.

Clarke, S. P., and N. E. Donaldson. 2008. "Nurse Staffing and Patient Care Quality and Safety. In *Patient Safety and Quality: An Evidence-Based Handbook for Nurses,* edited by R. G. Hughes. AHRQ Publication No. 08-0043. Rockville, MD: Agency for Healthcare Research and Quality. [Online publication; retrieved 2/13/11.] www.ncbi.nlm.nih.gov/books/NBK2676/http://www.ncbi.nlm.nih.gov/books/NBK2676/

Classen, D. C., R. C. Lloyd, L. Provost, F. A. Griffin, and R. Resar. 2008. "Development and Evaluation of the Institute for Healthcare Improvement Global Trigger Tool." *Journal of Patient Safety* 4 (3): 169–77.

Cleves, M. A., and W. E. Golden. 1996. "Assessment of HCFA's 1992 Medicare Hospital Information Report of Mortality Following Admission for Hip Arthroplasty." *Health Services Research* 31 (1): 39–48.

Cliff, B. 2010. "The Leadership Journey of Patient-Centered Care." *Frontiers of Health Services Management* 26 (4): 35–39.

Cockshut-Miller, L. (ed.). 2004. *Tracer Methodology: Tips and Strategies for Continuous Systems Improvement.* Oakbrook Terrace, IL: Joint Commission Resources.

Cohen, M. R. 1999. "One Hospital's Method of Applying Failure Mode and Effects Analysis." In *Medication Errors,* edited by M. R. Cohen, 4.1–4.4. Washington, DC: American Pharmaceutical Association.

Coles, G., B. Fuller, K. Kordquist, and A. Kongslie. 2005. "Using Failure Mode Effects and Criticality Analysis for High-Risk Processes at Three Community Hospitals." *The Joint Commission Journal on Quality and Patient Safety* 31 (3): 132–40.

Covey, S. 2004. *The Seven Habits of Highly Effective People: Powerful Lessons in Personal Change.* New York: Free Press.

Covey, S. R. 1990. *The Seven Habits of Highly Effective People.* New York: Simon and Schuster.

Critical Thinking Community. 2010. "Defining Critical Thinking." [Online information; retrieved 9/1/10.] www.criticalthinking.org/page.cfm?PageID=796&CategoryID=103#2424

Croteau, R. J. (ed.). 2010. *Root Cause Analysis in Health Care: Tools and Techniques.* Oakbrook Terrace, IL: Joint Commission Resources.

Culliton, B. J. 2006. "Extracting Knowledge from Science: A Conversation with Elias Zerhouni." *Health Affairs Web Exclusives Supplement* 25: W94–W103.

Dalrymple, J., and E. Drew. 2000. "Quality: On the Threshold or the Brink?" *Total Quality Management* 11 (4–6): 697–703.

Davis, S. M. 1982. "Transforming Organizations: The Key to Strategy Is Context." *Organizational Dynamics* 10 (3): 64–80.

Dean, J. W., and D. E. Bowen. 2000. "Management Theory and Total Quality: Improving Research and Practice Through Theory Development." In *The Quality Movement and Organization Theory,* edited by R. E. Cole and W. R. Scott. Thousand Oaks, CA: Sage Publications.

Deming, W. E. 2000. *Out of the Crisis,* 88. Cambridge, MA: The MIT Press.

Dictionary of Psychology Online. 2009a. s. v. "cognitive psychology." In *Oxford Reference Online.* [Online entry; retrieved 8/17/10.] www.oxfordreference.com.libproxy.lib.unc.edu/views/ENTRY .html?subview=Main&entry=t87.e1617

Dictionary of Psychology Online. 2009b. s. v. "schema." In *Oxford Reference Online.* [Online entry; retrieved 8/17/10.] www.oxfordreference.com.lib-proxy.lib.unc.edu/views/ENTRY.html?subview=Main&entry=t87.e7351.

Donabedian, A. 1980. *Explorations in Quality Assessment and Monitoring, Volume 1: The Definition of Quality and Approaches to Its Assessment.* Chicago: Health Administration Press.

Dorner, D. 1996. *The Logic of Failure: Recognizing and Avoiding Error in Complex Situations.* Reading, MA: Perseus Books.

Dugan, I. J. 2010. "Wrong-Way Financial Bets Have Hit Hard." *The Wall Street Journal,* July 10.

Encarta Online Dictionary. 2011. s. v. "pattern." [Online entry; retrieved 1/17/11.] http://encarta.msn.com/encnet/features/dictionary/ DictionaryResults.aspx?lextype=3&search=pattern%20

Evans, R. S., S. L. Pestotnik, D. C. Classen, T. P. Clemmer, L. K. Weaver, J. F. Orme, J. F. Lloyd, and J. P. Burke. 1998. "A Computer-Assisted Management Program for Antibiotics and Other Antiinfective Agents." *New England Journal of Medicine* 338 (4): 232–38.

Facione, P. A., N. C. Facione, C. A. F. Giancarlo, and S. W. Blohm. 2002. "Teaching for Thinking." [Online article; retrieved 9/2/10.] www.insightassessment.com/pdf_files/CT_Teaching_tips.pdf

Fischetti, M. 2001. "Drowning New Orleans." *Scientific American.* [Online article; retrieved 1/17/11.] www.scientificamerican.com/article .cfm?id=drowning-new-orleans-hurricane-prediction

Fisher, K. 2000. *Leading Self-Directed Work Teams: A Guide to Developing New Team Leadership Skills.* New York: McGraw-Hill.

Fitzgerald, J. F., P. S. Moore, and R. S. Dittus. 1988. "The Care of Elderly Patients with Hip Fracture. Changes Since Implementation of the Prospective Payment System." *New England Journal of Medicine* 319 (21): 1392–97.

Frampton, S., and C. Wahl. 2010. "What It Takes to Be Patient-Centered." *American Journal of Nursing*, Planetree, and Picker Institute Putting Patients First Webcast Series. [Online webinar; retrieved 8/22/10.] http://event.on24.com/r.htm?e=208531&s=1&k= 92675DC3302905F61799ECF13CFEA1F1

Frankl, V. E. 1962. *Man's Search for Meaning: An Introduction to Logotherapy.* Boston: Beacon Press.

Friis, R. H., and T. A. Sellers. 2009. *Epidemiology for Public Health Practice.* Sudbury, MA: Jones and Bartlett Publishers.

Fritz, R. 1996. *Corporate Tides: The Inescapable Laws of Organizational Structure.* San Francisco: Berrett-Koehler Publishers.

———. 1989. *The Path of Least Resistance: Learning to Become the Creative Force in Your Own Life.* New York: Ballantine.

Garibaldi, R. A. 1998. "Computers and the Quality of Care—A Clinician's Perspective." *New England Journal of Medicine* 338 (4): 259–60.

Georgopoulos, B. S., and F. C. Mann. 1962. *The Community General Hospital.* New York: The MacMillan Company.

Gibson, R., and J. P. Singh. 2003. *Wall of Silence: The Untold Story of the Medical Mistakes That Kill and Injure Millions of Americans.* Washington, DC: LifeLine Press.

Gilboy, N., P. Tanabe, D. A. Travers, A. M. Rosenau, and D. R. Eitel. 2005. *Emergency Severity Index, Version 4: Implementation Handbook.* AHRQ Publication No. 05-0046-2. Rockville, MD: Agency for Healthcare Research and Quality.

Giordano, L. A., M. N. Elliott, E. Goldstein, W. G. Lehrman, and P. A. Spencer. 2010. "Development, Implementation and Public Reporting of the HCAHPS Survey." *Medical Care* 67 (1): 27–37.

Gitlin, L. N., and K. J. Lyons. 2008. *Successful Grant Writing: Strategies for Health and Human Service Professionals.* New York: Springer Publishing Company.

Gold, J. 2011. "ACO is the Hottest Three Letter Word in Health Care." *Kaiser Health News*, Jan. 13. [Online information; retrieved 1/17/11.] www .kaiserhealthnews.org/Stories/2011/January/13/ACO-accountable-care-organization-FAQ.aspx

Goldratt, E. M. 1990. *The Haystack Syndrome: Sifting Information Out of the Data Ocean.* New York: North River Press, Inc.

Gordon, S. 2005. *Nursing Against the Odds: How Health Care Cost Cutting, Media Stereotypes and Medical Hubris Undermine Nurses and Patient Care.* Ithaca, NY: Cornell University Press.

Gosbee J. W. (ed.). 2005. *Using Human Factors Engineering to Improve Patient Safety.* Oakbrook Terrace, IL: Joint Commission Resources, Inc.

Goss, T., R. Pascale, and A. Athos. 1998. "The Reinvention Roller Coaster: Risking the Present for a Powerful Future." In *Harvard Business Review on Change*, 83–112. Boston: Harvard Business School Press.

Graham, M. 2002. "Is Sunshine the Best Disinfectant? The Promise and Problems of Environmental Disclosure." [Online information; retrieved 5/7/06.] www.brookings.edu/press/review/spring2002/graham.htm

Griffith, J. R., and K. R. White. 2005. "The Revolution in Hospital Management." *Journal of Healthcare Management* 50 (3): 170–90.

Gulliver, B., and D. Kelly. 2009. Unpublished paper, University of Utah, master student presentation.

Gurd, B., and T. Gao. 2008. "Lives in the Balance: An Analysis of the Balanced Scorecard (BSC) in Healthcare Organizations." *International Journal of Productivity & Performance Management* 57 (1): 6–21.

Guterman, S., K. Davis, K., Stremikis, and H. Drake. 2010. "Innovation in Medicare and Medicaid Will Be Central to Health Reform's Success." *Health Affairs* 29 (6): 1188–93.

Hanlan, M. 2004. *High Performance Teams: How to Make Them Work.* Westport, CT: Praeger Publishers.

Hanna, D. P. 1988. *Designing Organizations for High Performance.* Reading, MA: Addison Wesley Publishing Company.

Harrison, J. P., and L. Curran. 2009. "The Hospitalist Model: Does It Enhance Health Care Quality?" *Journal of Health Care Finance* 35 (3): 22–34.

HCAHPS. 2010. "HCAHPS Survey." [Online survey instrument; retrieved 7/8/2010.] http://hcahpsonline.org/Files/HCAHPS%20V6%200%20 Appendix%20A%20-%20HCAHPS%20Mail%20Survey%20Materials%20 (English)%202-16-2011.pdf

Healthy People. 2011. "About Healthy People: Introducing Healthy People 2020." [Online report; retrieved 1/30/11.] www.healthypeople.gov/ 2020/about/default.aspx

Heifetz, R. A. and D. L. Laurie. 2001. "The Work of Leadership." *Harvard Business Review* 79 (11): 131–40.

Helmreich, R. L. 1997. "Managing Human Error in Aviation." *Scientific American* 276 (5): 62–67.

Helmreich, R. L., A. C. Merritt, and J. A. Wilhelm. 1999. "The Evolution of Crew Resource Management Training in Commercial Aviation." *International Journal of Aviation Psychology* 9 (1): 19–32.

Hofmann, P. B. 2005. "Acknowledging and Examining Management Mistakes." In *Management Mistakes in Healthcare: Identification, Correction and Prevention*, edited by P. B. Hofmann and F. Perry, 3–27. Cambridge, UK: Cambridge University Press.

Holt, L., and M. Kysilka. 2006. *Instructional Patterns: Strategies for Maximizing Student Learning.* Thousand Oaks, CA: Sage Publications.

Horn, E., and J. Jacobi. 2006. "The Critical Care Clinical Pharmacist: Evolution of an Essential Team Member." *Critical Care Medicine* 34 (3S): S46–S51.

Houlihan, A. 2007. "The New Melting Pot: How to Effectively Lead Different Generations in the Workplace." *Supervision* 68 (9): 10–12.

Iezzoni, L. I. (ed.). 2003. *Risk Adjustment for Measuring Health Care Outcomes*, 3rd ed. Chicago: Health Administration Press.

Innovations Associates. 1995. "Systems Thinking: A Language for Learning and Action." Participant manual, version 95.4.1. Waltham, MA: Innovations Associates.

Institute for Healthcare Improvement (IHI). 2010. "Improvement Methods." [Online article; retrieved 4/5/11.] www.ihi.org/IHI/Topics/ Improvement/ImprovementMethods/HowToImprove

———. 2009. "Improving Your HCAHPS Score Through Patient-Centered Care." [Online program advertisement; published 12/1/09.] www.ihi .org/IHI/Programs/AudioAndWebPrograms/ExpeditionImproving HCAHPSScoreThroughPatientCenteredCare.htm

Institute of Medicine. 2001a. *Crossing the Quality Chasm: A New Health System for the 21st Century.* Washington, DC: National Academies Press.

———. 2001b. *Envisioning the National Health Care Quality Report,* edited by M. H. Hurtado, E. K. Swift, and J. M. Corrigan. Washington, DC: National Academies Press. [Online publication; released 3/30/01.] www .iom.edu/Reports/2001/Envisioning-the-National-Health-Care-Quality-Report.aspx

———. 1999. *To Err Is Human: Building a Safer Health System,* edited by L. T. Kohn, J. M. Corrigan, and M. S. Donaldson. Washington, DC: National Academies Press.

Isaac, T., A. M. Zaslavsky, P. D. Cleary, and B. E. Landon. 2010. "The Relationship Between Patients' Perception of Care and Measures of Hospital Quality and Safety." *Health Services Research* 45 (4): 1024–40.

Jencks, S. F., T. Cuerdon, D. R. Burwen, B. Fleming, P. M. Houck, A. E. Kussmaul, D. S. Nilasena, D. L. Ordin, and D. R. Arday. 2000. "Quality of Medical Care Delivered to Medicare Beneficiaries: A Profile at State and National Levels." *JAMA* 284 (13): 1670–76.

Jencks, S. F., E. D. Huff, and T. Cuerdon. 2003. "Change in the Quality of Care Delivered to Medicare Beneficiaries, 1998–1999 to 2000–2001." *JAMA* 289 (3): 305–12.

Jha, A. K., E. J. Oray, J. Zheng, and A. M. Epstein. 2008. "Patients' Perception of Hospital Care in the United States." *The New England Journal of Medicine* 359 (18): 1921–31.

Jha, A. K., Z. Li, E. J. Orav, and A. M. Epstein. 2005. "Care in U.S. Hospitals—The Hospital Quality Alliance Program." *The New England Journal of Medicine* 353 (3): 265–74.

Jiang, J. H., C. Lockee, K. Bass, and I. Fraser. 2008. "Board Engagement in Quality: Findings of a Survey for Hospital and System Leaders." *Journal of Healthcare Management* 53 (2): 121–35.

The Joint Commission. 2010a. *2010 Comprehensive Accreditation Manual—Electronic Edition.* [Online information; retrieved 8/17/2010.] http:// amp.jcrinc.com

———. 2010b. "Facts About Unannounced Surveys." [Online fact sheet; retrieved 10/16/2010.] www.jointcommission.org/AboutUs/Fact_ Sheets/unannounced.htm

———. 2010c. *Improving America's Hospitals: The Joint Commission's Annual Report on Quality and Safety.* [Online information; retrieved 10/15/2010.] www.jointcommission.org/NR/rdonlyres/D60136A2-6A59-4009-A6F3-04E2FF230991/0/2010_Annual_Report.pdf

———. 2010d. "National Patient Safety Goals." [Online information; retrieved 7/1/10.] www.jointcommission.org/patientsafety/ nationalpatientsafetygoals/

———. 2010e. "National Patient Safety Goals Universal Protocol." [Online information; retrieved 7/4/2010.] www.jointcommission.org/

NR/rdonlyres/868C9E07-037F-433D-8858-0D5FAA4322F2/0/
July2010NPSGs_Scoring_HAP2.pdf

———. 2010f. s. v. "sentinel event." *Glossary of Terms.* [Online entry; retrieved 10/8/2010.] www.jointcommission.org/SentinelEvents/se_glossary.htm

———. 2010g. Website. [Online information; retrieved 10/6/2010.] www.jointcommission.org

———. 2009a. "Facts About the National Patient Safety Goals." [Online information; retrieved 7/8/2010.] www.jointcommission.org/PatientSafety/NationalPatientSafetyGoals/npsg_facts.htm

———. 2009b. "A Framework for a Root Cause Analysis and Action Plan in Response to a Sentinel Event." [Online information; retrieved 8/29/10.] www.jointcommission.org/SentinelEvents/Forms/

———. 2007. "Sentinel Event Policy." [Online information; retrieved 8/29/10.] www.jointcommission.org/NR/rdonlyres/F84F9DC6-A5DA-490F-A91F-A9FCE26347C4/0/SE_chapter_july07.pdf

———. 2005. "The Fact on Fiction: Organizations Do Not Need to Prepare for Their Next Survey; They Need to Prepare for Their Next Patient." *Joint Commission Perspectives* 25 (2): 7. [Online edition; retrieved 6/21/10.] www.jcrinc.com/The-Joint-Commission-Perspectives

The Joint Commission and Centers for Medicare & Medicaid Services. 2010. *Specifications Manual for National Hospital Inpatient Quality Measures.* [Online information; retrieved 10/20/2010.] www.jointcommission.org/PerformanceMeasurement/PerformanceMeasurement/Current+NHQM+Manual.htm

Joint Commission and Joint Commission Resources. 2004. "Special Report: JCAHO Shared Visions–New Pathways." *Joint Commission Perspectives, The Official Joint Commission Newsletter* 24 (1): 1–27.

Joint Commission Resources. 2003. "Shared Visions–New Pathways: An Innovative Approach to Patient Safety and Quality Improvement." [Video.] Oakbrook Terrace, IL: Joint Commission.

Jones, C. B. 2008. "Revisiting Turnover Costs: Adjusting for Inflation." *Journal of Nursing Administration* 38 (1): 11–18.

Journal of the American Medical Association (JAMA). 2010. "JAMA Evidence: Using Evidence to Improve Care." [Online article; retrieved 9/27/10.] www.jamaevidence.com

Juran, J. M. 1989. *Juran on Leadership for Quality: An Executive Handbook.* New York: The Free Press.

Kaboli, P. J., A. B. Hoth, B. J. McClimon, and J. L. Schnipper. 2006. "Clinical Pharmacists and Inpatient Medical Care: A Systematic Review." *Archives of Internal Medicine* 166: 955–96.

Kaiser Family Foundation. 2011. *State Health Facts.* [Online information; retrieved 2/12/2011.] www.statehealthfacts.org/comparemaptable.jsp?ind=54&cat=2

Kaiser Family Foundation (producer). 2005. "Medicare and Medicaid at 40." [Online video; retrieved 6/23/10.] www.kff.org/medicaid/40years.cfm

Kaplan, R. S., and D. P. Norton. 2007. "Using the Balanced Scorecard as a Strategic Management System." *Harvard Business Review* 85 (7/8): 150–61.

————. 2005. "The Balanced Scorecard: Measures that Drive Performance." *Harvard Business Review* 83 (7/8): 172–80.

Kauffman, D. R. 1980. *Systems One: An Introduction to Systems Thinking.* Minneapolis, MN: Future Systems, Inc.

Kelly, D. 2009a. "Creating and Leading Error-Free Management Systems." Seminar presented by the American College of Healthcare Executives, Atlanta, GA, September 16–17.

————. 2009b. "Quality Assurance and Performance Improvement." Presented at the American College of Healthcare Executives Board of Governors Examination Review Course, Chicago, May 13.

————. 2009c. "Response to: Donald M. Berwick 'Confessions of an Extremist.'" *Health Affairs* 28 (4): w555–w565.

————. 1999. "Systems Thinking: A Tool for Organizational Diagnosis in Healthcare." In *Making It Happen: Stories from Inside the New Workplace.* Waltham, MA: Pegasus Communications, Inc.

————. 1998. "Reframing Beliefs About Work and Change Processes in Redesigning Laboratory Services." *Joint Commission Journal on Quality Improvement* 24 (9): 154–67.

Kelly, D. L., and S. L. Pestotnik. 1998. "Using Causal Loop Diagrams to Facilitate Double Loop Learning in the Healthcare Delivery Setting." Unpublished manuscript.

Kelly, D. L., S. L. Pestotnik, M. C. Coons, and J. W. Lelis. 1997. "Reengineering a Surgical Service Line: Focusing on Core Process Improvement." *American Journal of Medical Quality* 12 (2): 120–29.

Kelly, D. L., and N. Short. 2006. "Exploring Assumptions About Teams." *Joint Commission Journal on Quality and Patient Safety* 32 (2): 109–12.

Kenagy, J. W., D. M. Berwick, and M. F. Shore. 1999. "Service Quality in Health Care." *Journal of the American Medical Association* 281 (7): 661–65.

Kok, G., N. H. Gottlieb, M. Commers, and C. Smerecnik. 2008. "The Ecological Approach in Health Promotion Programs: A Decade Later." *American Journal of Health Promotion* 22 (6): 437–42.

Kouzes, J. M., and B. Z. Posner. 2007. *The Leadership Challenge,* 4th ed. San Francisco: Jossey-Bass.

Kritchevsky, S. B., and B. P. Simmons. 1995. "The Tools of Quality Improvement: CQI Versus Epidemiology." *Infection Control and Hospital Epidemiology* 16: 499–502.

Langley, G. J., K. M. Nolan, T. W. Nolan, C. L. Norman, and L. P. Provost. 1996. *The Improvement Guide: A Practical Approach to Enhancing Organizational Performance.* San Francisco: Jossey-Bass.

The Leapfrog Group. 2010. "Factsheet." [Online information; retrieved 7/8/2010.] www.leapfroggroup.org/media/file/FactSheet_LeapfrogGroup.pdf

Leavitt, M. O. 2006. *Report to Congress: Improving the Medicare Quality Improvement Organization Program—Response to the Institute of Medicine Study.* [Online report; retrieved 10/9/2010.] www.cms.gov/QualityImprovementOrgs/downloads/QIO_Improvement_RTC_fnl.pdf

Leonard, D., and S. Straus. 1997. "Putting Your Company's Whole Brain to Work." *Harvard Business Review* 75 (4): 110–19.

Lloyd, R. 2010. "Helping Leaders Blink Correctly." *Healthcare Executive* 25 (3): 88–91.

Lohr, K. N. (ed.). 1990. *Medicare: A Strategy for Quality Assurance.* Washington, DC: National Academies Press.

Longest, B. B. 2010. *Health Policymaking in the United States,* 5th ed. Chicago: Health Administration Press.

Lopez, L., L. S. Hicks, A. P. Cohen, S. McKean, and J. S. Weissman. 2009. "Hospitalists and the Quality of Care in Hospitals." *Archives of Internal Medicine* 169 (15): 1389–94.

Mason, K. D., J. K. Leavitt, and M. W. Chaffee. 2007. "Policy & Politics: A Framework for Action." In *Policy & Politics in Nursing and Health Care,* edited by K. D. Mason, J. K. Leavitt, and M. W. Chaffee, 1–20. St. Louis, MO: Elsevier.

McCormack, B., A. Kitson, G. Harvey, J. Rycroft-Malone, A. Titchen, and K. Seers. 2002. "Getting Evidence into Practice: The Meaning of 'Context.'" *Journal of Advanced Nursing* 38 (1): 94–104.

McHugh, M., A. Garman, A. McAlearney, P. Song, and M. Harrison. 2010. *Using Workforce Practices to Drive Quality Improvement: A Guide for Hospitals.* Chicago: Health Research & Educational Trust.

McNeil, J. P., D. Brown, D. Howard, B. McClure, and G. R. Weedon. 2002. "Sterilization Protects Animals and You." Presentation to the University of North Carolina at Chapel Hill Management Academy for Public Health, April 25.

Medline Plus Merriam-Webster Medical Dictionary. 2011. s. v. "pharmacotherapeutics." [Online entry; retrieved 1/17/11.] www.merriam-webster.com/medlineplus/pharmacotherapeutics

Merriam-Webster Dictionary Online. 2011. s. v. "policy." [Online entry; retrieved 2/28/11.] www.merriam-webster.com

———. 2010a. s. v. "context." [Online entry; retrieved 11/3/10.] www.merriam-webster.com/

———. 2010b. s. v. "manage." [Online entry; retrieved 12/1/10.] www.merriam-webster.com/dictionary/manage

———. 2010c. s. v. "team." [Online entry; retreived 10/1/10.] www.merriam-webster.com

Merrill, R. M., and T. C. Timmreck. 2006. *Introduction to Epidemiology,* 4th ed. Sudbury, MA: Jones and Bartlett Publishers.

Myers, I. B., L. K. Kirby, and K. D. Myers. 1998. *Introduction to Type: A Guide to Understanding Your Results on the Myers-Briggs Type Indicator.* Palo Alto, CA: Consulting Psychologists Press.

Nadler, G., and S. Hibino. 1994. *Breakthrough Thinking: The Seven Principles of Creative Problem Solving.* Rocklin, CA: Prima Publishing.

National Center for Biotechnology Information (NCBI). 2004. "One Size Does Not Fit All: The Promise of Pharamcogenomics." [Online article; revised 3/31/04.] www.ncbi.nlm.nih.gov/About/primer/pharm.html

National Committee for Quality Assurance (NCQA). Website. 2010. [Online information; retrieved 10/6/2010.] www.ncqa.org/

National Institute of Standards and Technology. 2011. *2011–2012 Health Care Criteria for Performance Excellence.* Washington, DC: National Institute of Standards and Technology. [Online information; retrieved 1/30/11.] www.nist.gov/baldrige/publications/hc_criteria.cfm

National Quality Forum. 2004. *National Voluntary Consensus Standards for Nursing-Sensitive Care: An Initial Performance Measure Set.* [Online information; retrieved 10/2/10.] www.qualityforum.org/Projects/n-r/ Nursing-Sensitive_Care_Initial_Measures/Nursing_Sensitive_Care__ Initial_Measures.aspx

National Snow and Ice Data Center (NSIDC). 2011. "Quick Facts." [Online entry; retrieved 1/17/2011.] http://nsidc.org/glaciers/quickfacts.html

Nelson E. C., P. B. Batalden, T. P. Hubor, J. K. Johnson, M. M. Godfrey, L. A. Headrick, and J. H. Wasson. 2007. "Success Characteristics of High-Performing Microsystems." In *Quality by Design: A Clinical Microsystem Approach,* edited by E. C. Nelson, P. B. Batalden, and M. M. Godfrey. San Francisco: Jossey-Bass.

Nelson, E. C., J. J. Mohr, P. B. Batalden, and S. K. Plume. 1996. "Improving Healthcare, Part 1: The Clinical Value Compass." *Joint Commission Journal on Quality Improvement* 22 (4): 243–58.

Norman, D. A. 2002. *Design of Everyday Things.* New York: Perseus Books.

Oleske, D. M. 2009. *Epidemiology and the Delivery of Health Care Services: Methods and Applications.* New York: Springer.

Patient Protection and Affordable Care Act of 2010, Pub. L. 111-148 (2010).

Petzinger, T. 1998. "Nurses Discover the Healing Power of Customer Service" *Wall Street Journal,* Feb. 27, B1.

The Picker Institute. Website. 2010. [Online information; retrieved 8/22/10.] www.pickerinstitute.org

Pierce, J. C. 2000. "The Paradox of Physicians and Administrators in Healthcare Organizations." *Healthcare Management Review* 25 (1): 7–28.

President's Advisory Committee on Consumer Protection and Quality in the Health Care Industry. 1998. "Quality First: Better Health Care for All Americans." [Online information; retrieved 10/14/2010.] www.hcquality-commission.gov/final/

Pronovost, P. J., D. C. Angus, T. Dorman, K. A. Robinson, T. T. Dremsizov, and T. L. Young. 2002. "Physician Staffing Patterns and Clinical Outcomes in Critically Ill Patients: A Systematic Review." *JAMA* 288: 2151–62.

Public Health Accreditation Board (PHAB). Website. 2010. [Online information; retrieved 10/7/2010.] www.phaboard.org

Reason, J. 1997. *Managing the Risks of Organizational Accidents.* Hampshire, UK: Ashgate Publishing Company.

———. 1995. "Understanding Adverse Events: Human Factors." *Quality and Safety in Healthcare* 4: 80–89.

———. 1990. *Human Error.* Cambridge, UK: Cambridge University Press.

Reed, P. 2001. "Introduction to Social Behavior in Public Health." Course lecture at the Department of Health Behavior and Health Education, University of North Carolina at Chapel Hill, School of Public Health.

Reiling, J. G., B. L. Knutzen, and M. Stocklein. 2003. "FMEA—The Cure for Medical Errors." *Quality Progress* 36 (8): 67–71.

Reiman T., E. Pietikäinen, and P. Oedewald. 2010. "Multilayered Approach to Patient Safety Culture." *Quality and Safety in Healthcare* online. doi: 10.1136/qsh.2008.029793. [Online article; retrieved 8/24/10.] http://qshc.bmj.com

Roberts, K. 1990. "Some Characteristics of One Type of High Reliability Organization." *Organizational Science* 1: 160–76.

Roberts, K., and R. Bea. 2001. "Must Accidents Happen? Lessons from High Reliability Organizations."*Academy of Management Executives* 15 (3): 70–78.

Rogers, E. M. 1995. *Diffusion of Innovations.* New York: The Free Press.

Rooney, A. L., and P. R. Ostenburg. 1999. *Licensure, Accreditation, and Certification: Approaches to Health Service Quality.* Bethesda, MD: Quality Assurance Project. [Online white paper; retrieved 10/4/10.] www.qaproject.org/pubs/PDFs/accredmon.pdf

Roper, W. L., W. Winkenwerder, G. M. Hackbarth, and H. Krakauer. 1988. "Effectiveness in Health Care: An Initiative to Evaluate and Improve Medical Practice." *New England Journal of Medicine* 319 (18): 1197–202.

Rose, G. 2001. "Sick Individuals and Sick Populations." *International Journal of Epidemiology* 30: 427–32.

Sammer, C. E., K. Lykens, K. P. Singh, D. A. Mains, and N. A. Lackan. 2010. *Journal of Nursing Scholarship* 42 (2): 156–65.

Scholtes, P. R., B. L. Joiner, and B. J. Streibel. 2003. *The Team Handbook,* 3rd ed. Madison, WI: Oriel Inc.

Scott, R. A. 2003. *Organizations: Rational, Natural, and Open Systems,* 5th ed. Upper Saddle River, NJ: Prentice Hall.

Senders, J. W., and S. J. Senders. 1999. "Failure Mode and Effects Analysis in Medicine." In *Medication Errors,* edited by M. R. Cohen, 3.1–3.8. Washington, DC: American Pharmaceutical Association.

Senge, P. M. 2006. *The Fifth Discipline: The Art and Practice of the Learning Organization.* New York: Doubleday Currency.

———. 1990. *The Fifth Discipline: The Art and Practice of the Learning Organization.* New York: Doubleday Currency.

Shorr, A. S. 2007. "The Role of the Chief Executive Officer in Maximizing Patient Safety." *Healthcare Executive* 22 (2): 20–25.

Shortell, S. M., and A. D. Kaluzny. 2006. *Health Care Management: Organization Design and Behavior,* 5th ed. Albany, NY: Delmar Thomson Learning.

Shortell, S. M., J. L. O'Brien, J. M. Carman, R. W. Foster, E. F. X. Hughes, H. Boerstler, and E. J. O'Connor. 1995. "Assessing the Impact of Continuous Quality Improvement/Total Quality Management: Concept Versus Implementation." *Healthcare Research* 30 (2): 377–99.

Shortell, S. M., and S. J. Singer. 2008. "Improving Patient Safety by Taking Systems Seriously." *JAMA* 299 (4): 445–47.

Shortell, S. M., T. G. Rundall, and J. Hsu. 2007. "Improving Patient Care by Linking Evidence-Based Medicine and Evidence-Base Management." *Journal of the American Medical Association* 298 (6): 673–76.

Skyve, P. M. 2009. "Leadership in Healthcare Organizations: A Guide to Joint Commission Leadership Standards." A Governance Institute Whitepaper. [Online article; retrieved 8/24/10.] www.jointcommission.org/NR/rdonlyres/48366FFD-DB16-4C91-98F3-46C552A18D2A/0/WP_Leadership_Standards.pdf

Smith, M. 2002. "Quality Measurement in Healthcare: The Role of Public Reporting." University of North Carolina at Chapel Hill, School of Public Health Program on Health Outcomes, 2002 Spring Seminar Series, March 27.

Smith, R. 2000. *The Seven Levels of Change: The Guide to Innovation in the World's Largest Corporations.* Arlington, TX: The Summit Publishing Group.

Solberg, L. I. 2000a. "Incentivising, Facilitating and Implementing an Office Tobacco Cessation System." *Tobacco Control* 9 (Suppl 1): i37–41.

———. 2000b. "Lessons from Experienced Guideline Implementers: Attend to Many Factors and Use Multiple Strategies." *Joint Commission Journal on Quality Improvement* 26 (4): 171–88.

Spath, P. L. 2003. "Using Failure Mode and Effects Analysis to Improve Patient Safety." *Association of Operating Room Nurses Journal* 78: 16–37.

Starr, P. 1982. *The Social Transformation of American Medicine: The Rise of a Sovereign Profession and the Making of a Vast Industry.* Reading, MA: The Perseus Books Group.

Sterman, J. D. 2000. *Business Dynamics: Systems Thinking and Modeling for a Complex World.* Boston: Irwin McGraw-Hill.

Stern, A. M., and H. Markel. 2005. "The History of Vaccines and Immunization: Familiar Patterns, New Challenges." *Health Affairs* 24 (3): 611–21.

Stokols, D. 2000. "The Social Ecological Paradigm of Wellness Promotion." In *Promoting Human Wellness: New Frontiers for Research, Practice and Policy,* edited by M. D. Jamner and D. Stokols, 21–37. Los Angeles: University of California Press.

Tagg, J. 2007. "Double-Loop Learning in Higher Education." *Change* 9 (4): 36–41.

Tang, N., J. M. Eisenberg, and G. S. Meyer. 2004. "The Roles of Government in Improving Health Care Quality and Safety." *Joint Commission Journal on Quality and Safety* 30 (4): 47–55.

Taylor, B. B., E. R. Marcantonio, O. Pagovich, A. Carbo, M. Bergmann, R. B. Davis, D. W. Bates, R. S. Phillips, and S. N. Weingart. 2008. *Medical Care* 46 (2): 224–28.

Tunis, S. R., J. Benner, and M. McClellan. 2010. "Comparative Effectiveness Research: Policy Context, Methods Development and Research Infrastructure." *Statistics in Medicine* 29 (18): 1963–76.

US Department of Health and Human Service (HHS). 2010. Explanations of Process of Care Measures." [Online information; retrieved 7/4/2010.] www.hospitalcompare.hhs.gov/Hospital/Static/ConsumerInformation_tabset.asp?activeTab=2&Language=English&version=default&subTab=4

————. 2000. *Healthy People 2010: Understanding and Improving Health, 2nd edition.* [Online publication; retrieved 10/16/2010.] www.healthypeople.gov/Document/html/uih/uih_2.htm#deter

Viaene, S., and J. Willems. 2007. "Corporate Performance Management: Beyond Dashboards and Scorecards." *Journal of Performance Management* 20 (1): 13–32.

Waldman, J. D., F. Kelly, S. Arora, and H. L. Smith. 2010. "The Shocking Cost of Turnover in Healthcare." *Healthcare Management Review* 35 (3): 206–21.

Weick, K. E. 1984. "Small Wins: Redefining the Scale of Social Problems." *American Psychologist* 39 (1): 40–49.

Weisbord, M. R., and S. Janoff. 2010. *Future Search: Getting the Whole System in the Room for Vision, Commitment and Action,* 3rd ed. San Francisco: Berret-Koehler Publishers.

Wheatley, M. J. 1994. Self-Organizing Systems: The New Science of Change. Kelner-Rogers and Wheatley, Inc. Conference Proceedings, Deer Valley, Utah, October 17–19.

Wheeler, D. J. 2000. *Understanding Variation: The Key to Managing Chaos,* 2nd ed. Knoxville, TN: SPC Press.

Wilmington Morning Star. 2002. "Saving Pets and Taxpayers." Jan. 7, 6A.

World Health Organization. 2010. "Safe Surgery Saves Lives." [Online article; retrieved 6/22/10.] www.who.int/patientsafety/safesurgery/en/index.html

————. 2009. *A Guide to the Implementation of the WHO Multimodal Hand Hygiene Improvement Strategy.* [Online article; retrieved 10/31/10.] www.who.int/gpsc/5may/tools/en/

Yokoe, D. S., and D. Classen. 2008. "Improving Patient Safety Through Infection Control: A New Healthcare Imperative." *Infection Control and Hospital Epidemiology* 29: S3–S11.

Zhan, C., B. Friedman, A. Mosso, and P. Pronovost. 2006. "Medicare Payment for Selected Adverse Events: Building the Business Case for Investing In Patient Safety." *Health Affairs* 25 (5): 1386–93.

INDEX

ABOUT THE AUTHOR

Diane L. Kelly, DrPH, MBA, RN, is an expert in quality and performance excellence in healthcare delivery and public health organizations, international management development, organizational development in rural settings and underserved populations, and leadership development. Dr. Kelly's experience in healthcare organizations spans more than 30 years. Her diverse practice experience includes a not-for-profit integrated care system, academic medical centers, a for-profit community hospital, and a quality improvement organization. In addition, Dr. Kelly has consulted with more than 100 hospitals and health services organizations in the United States (including Native American healthcare facilities and numerous rural and frontier hospitals), in Central and Eastern Europe, and in Bermuda. Dr. Kelly served as a member of the board of examiners for the Baldrige Performance Excellence Program from 1999 to 2001, including the first year that healthcare organizations were eligible to apply for the national award. She served as an active member of the editorial advisory board for the *Joint Commission Journal for Quality and Safety* from 2004 to 2008. As the author of numerous peer-reviewed articles, Dr. Kelly's work has also been featured in the *Wall Street Journal.* Dr. Kelly maintains faculty responsibilities at the University of North Carolina at Chapel Hill Gillings School of Global Public Health in the Public Health Leadership Program; at Duke University School of Nursing; and at Weber State University Health Administration Services Program. Formerly, Dr. Kelly served as faculty for the University of North Carolina Management Academy for Public Health and as a faculty consultant for Project HOPE.